HIGH PROTEIN MEALS IN MINUTES

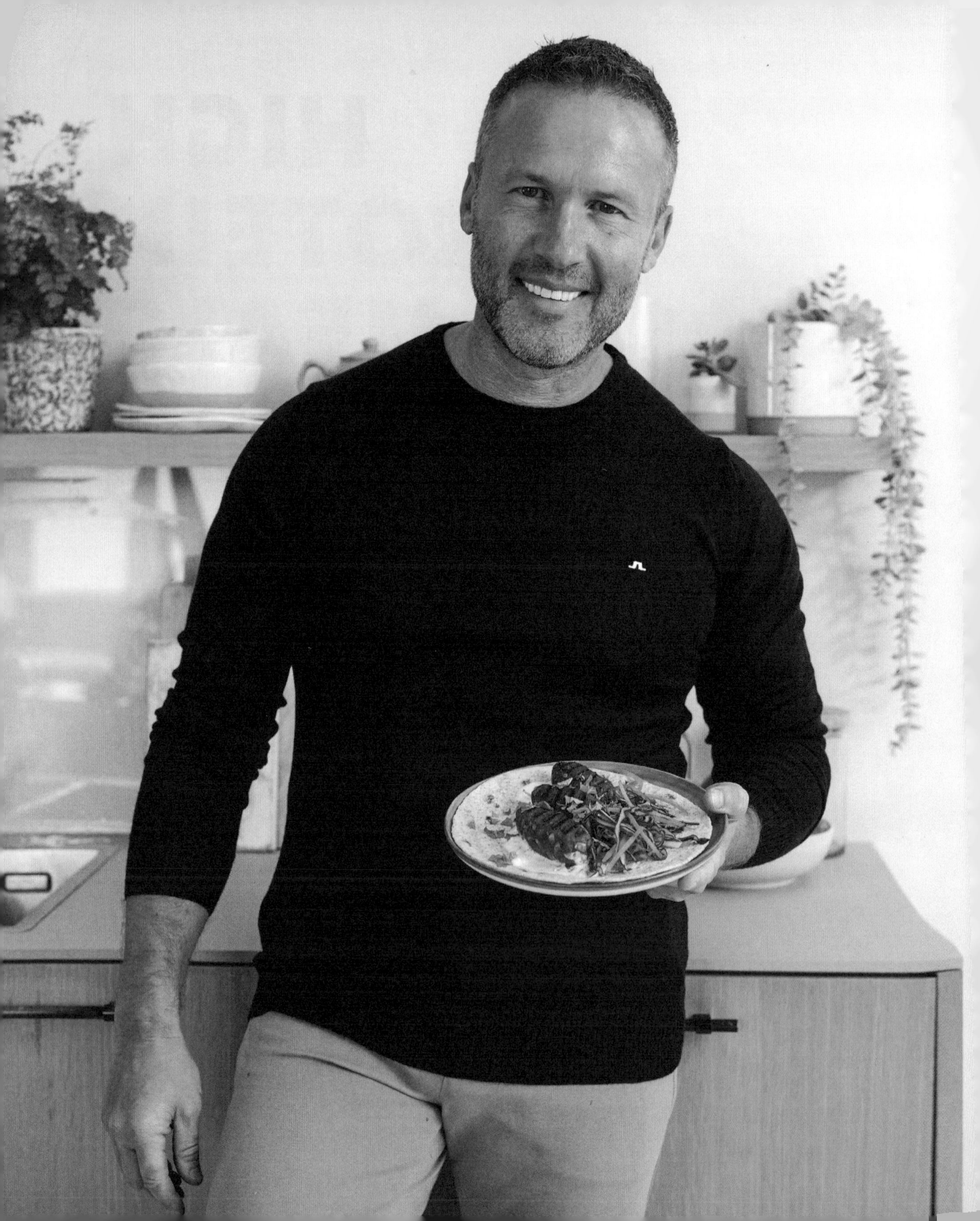

HIGH PROTEIN MEALS IN MINUTES

SCOTT HARRISON

Photography by David Cummings

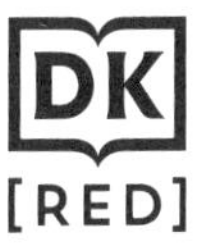

CONTENTS

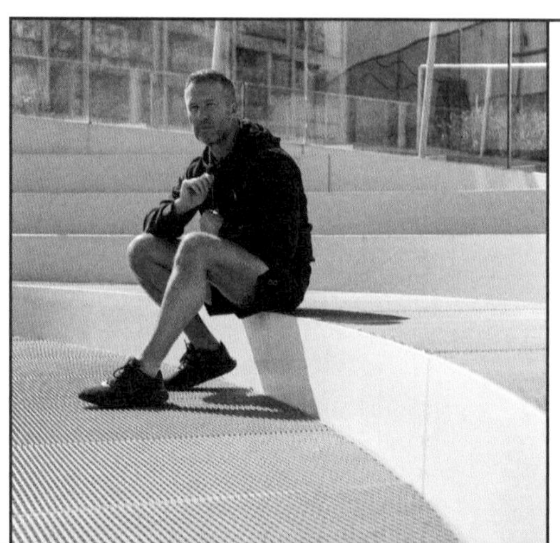

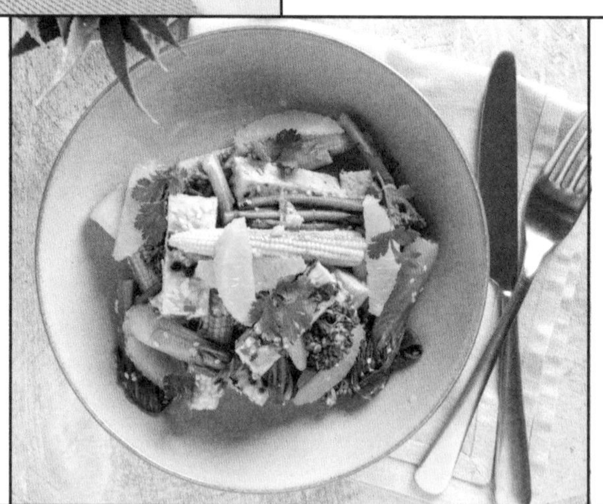

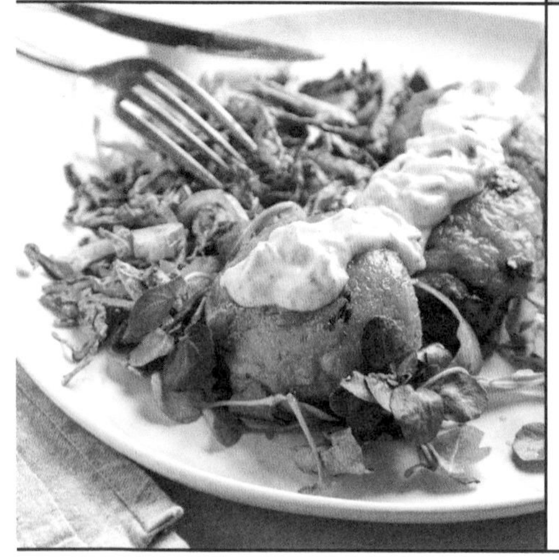

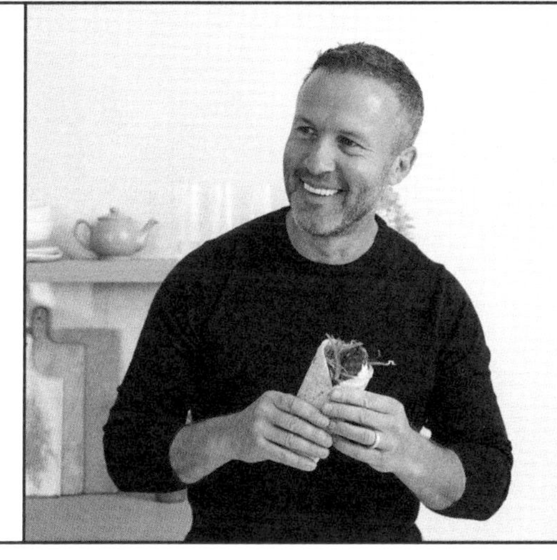

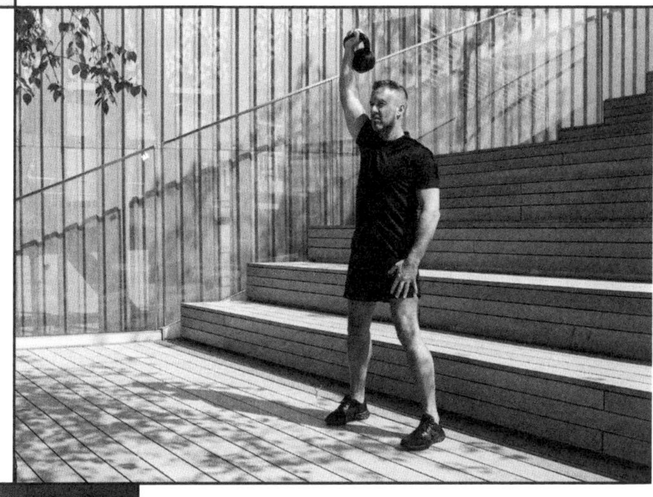

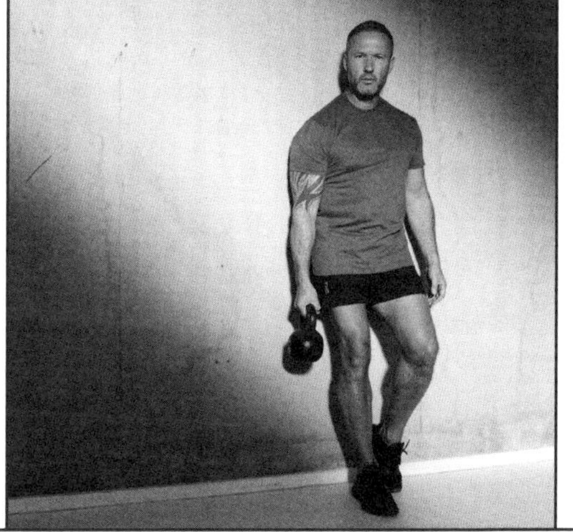

HEY FRIENDS . . .

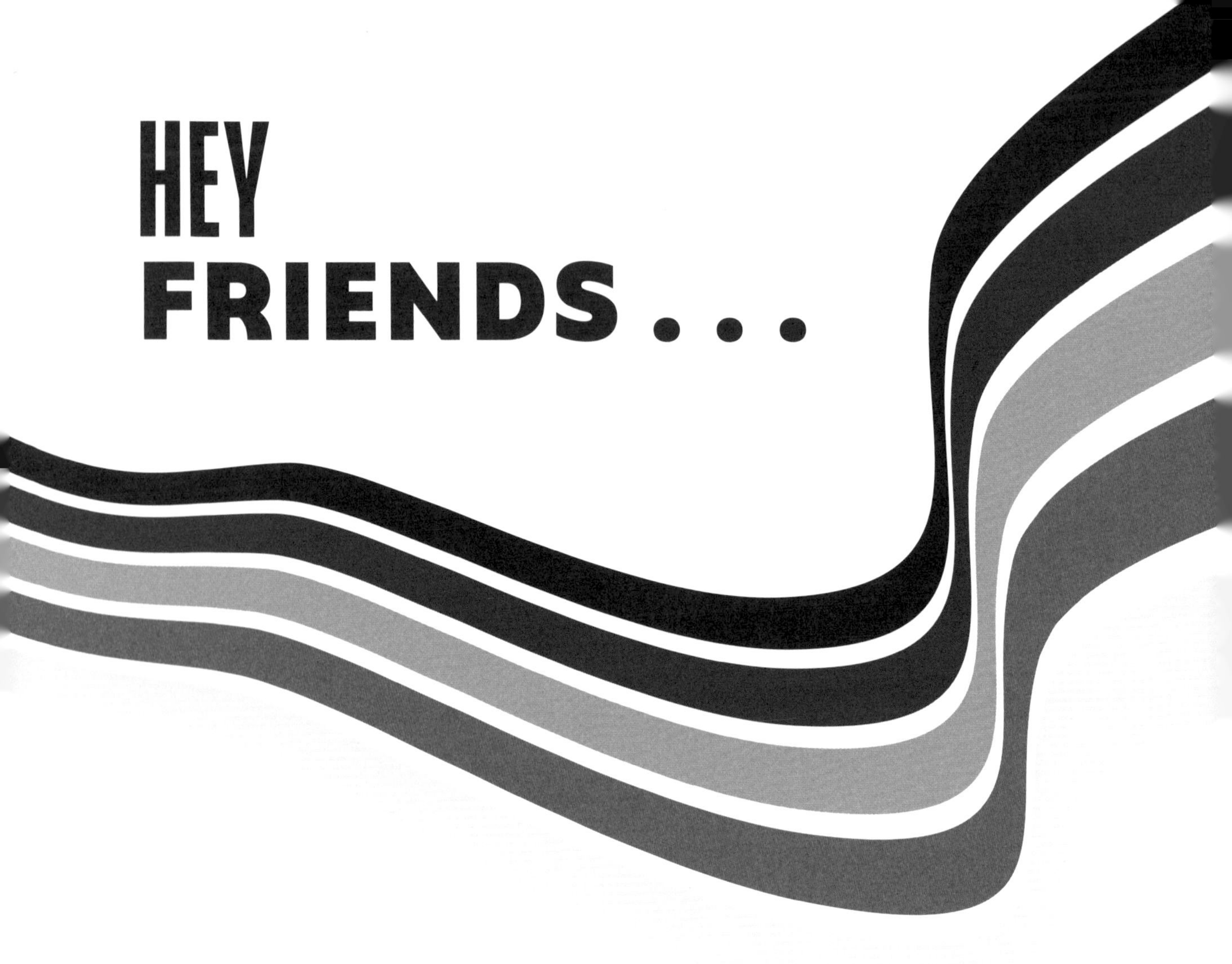

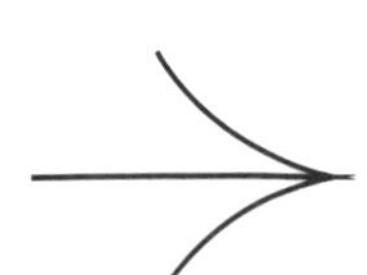

Welcome! To all those new to us looking to change their life for the better. AND... welcome back to all my friends who are already familiar with *Eat Your Way to a Six Pack*, I applaud your commitment to your health and wellbeing, what a much happier life it is, eh? It's fantastic to see you stepping onto this transformative journey, mirroring the exact path I myself embarked on many years ago.

They say abs are made in the kitchen, and I'm here to vouch for that! How many of you battle those irresistible cravings? How many diets have you experimented with, only to witness fleeting outcomes? If you're nodding along, you've walked the same path as me. But here's the truth – it's not merely about a temporary solution. It's about embracing vitality, energy, genuine happiness from within and changing your relationship with food, drink, and yourself. I'm no stranger to succumbing to the occasional temptation, but I've learned firsthand that my health outweighs any indulgence, meaning sometimes we have to tip the balance and switch what we think is pleasure for true happiness.

Within these pages, you will see that I've crafted an array of delectable recipes, easily adaptable for all diet preferences to help change your life and break free from your debilitating yo-yoing for good! From quick snacks to fuel your body, to meals you can share with friends, there's something for everyone. And in each recipe, there's an emphasis on balance.

You will also see in this book, I delve deeper into the "why" and "how" behind The Six Pack Revolution. From eating six times a day, why we don't focus on calories, to the rules of the hand; and balancing your hormones through food and exercise – this book serves as your guide and your motivator. Take the time to absorb its insights, and to find your mojo within the simplicity of your new lifestyle. Let the success story of myself and others inspire and empower you to create a success story of your own. Together, let's embark on a journey worth remembering.

As a modern renaissance man, my life's dedication is twofold: firstly, to my beautiful family, and secondly, to empowering others to reach their full potential. From serving as a fitness, nutrition and mindset expert to fulfilling roles as a life coach, motivational speaker, entrepreneur, and black belt karate instructor, I've worn many hats on this journey of empowerment. And now, as a proclaimed best-selling author, I continue to embrace every opportunity to uplift and inspire those around me.

I'm not just your teacher or health expert – I'm your guide, your mentor, and most of all, your biggest supporter.

Let's uplift and inspire! Join me on this unforgettable journey. Trust the process, and let's uncover your best self and truly live the amazing benefits of how your body and mind should feel. Ready? Let's make it happen!

Much love *Scotty* xxxx

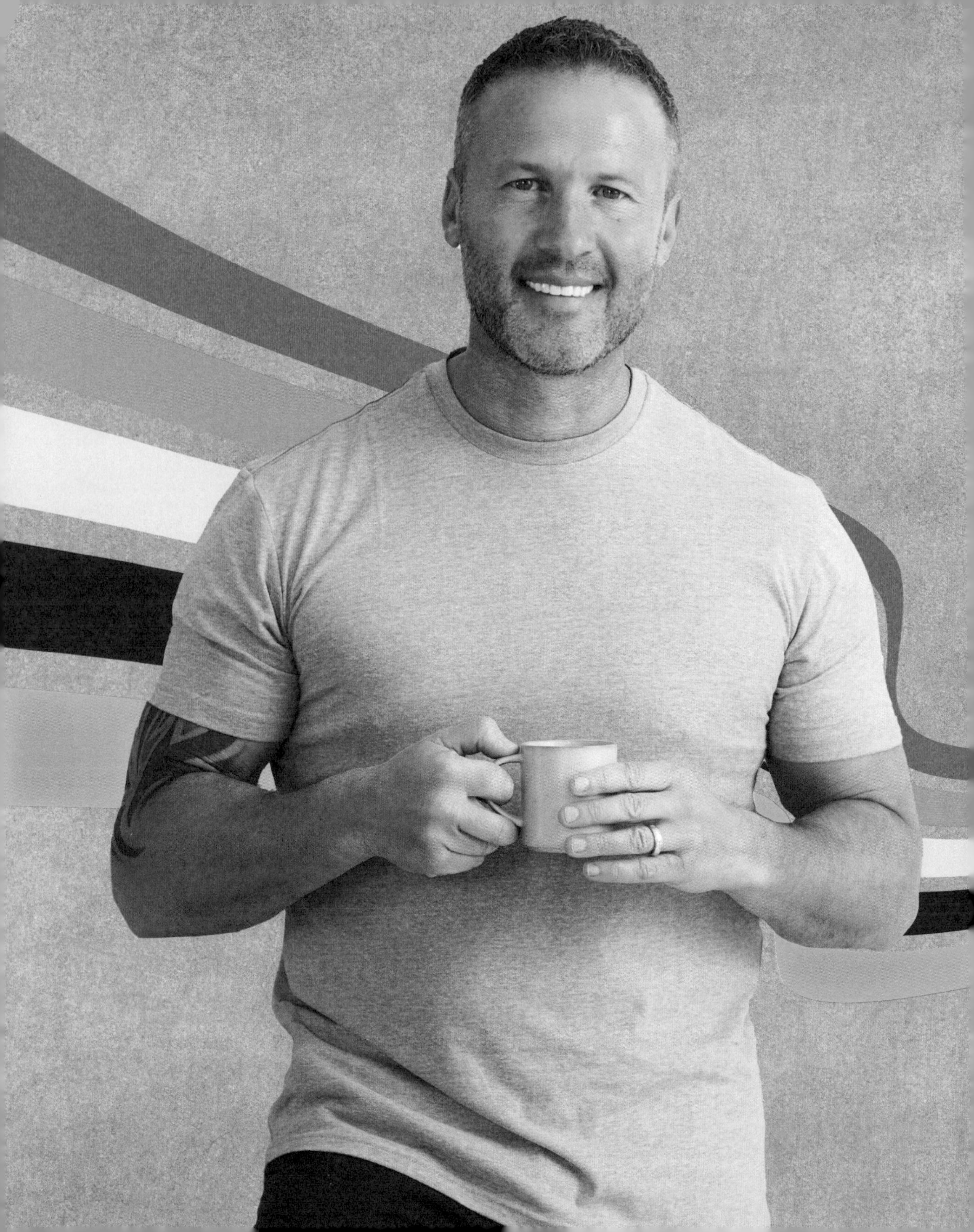

THE PROTEIN PLAN

Chapter 1

WHAT IS THE PROTEIN PLAN?

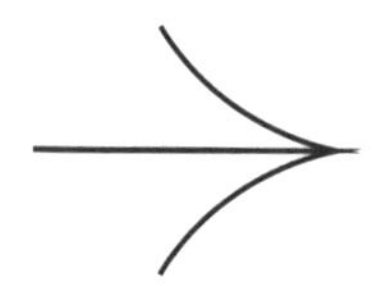

Extending the Six Pack Revolution to your kitchen, *High Protein Meals in Minutes* offers practical, time-saving meals and clear guidance to help you live a healthier and happier lifestyle. This book makes it easy for everyone to access delicious, high-protein recipes that can be prepared quickly. Protein is a crucial part of every meal because it helps repair tissues, build muscle, and support metabolic functions. It keeps you fuller for longer, aiding weight management and reducing unhealthy snacking.

Designed to save you time, I give you tips on how to batch-cook and focus on eating healthy, well-balanced, and delicious food. You'll find a variety of like-for-like swaps to cater to different dietary preferences so you can easily switch from lean meats, like chicken and turkey, to plant-based proteins, like soya (soy) and Quorn. These quick, adaptable recipes ensure every meal is full of flavour, high in protein, and easy to prepare, making healthy eating both simple and enjoyable.

Combining the recipes with the exercises that follow will help you get the results you're after.

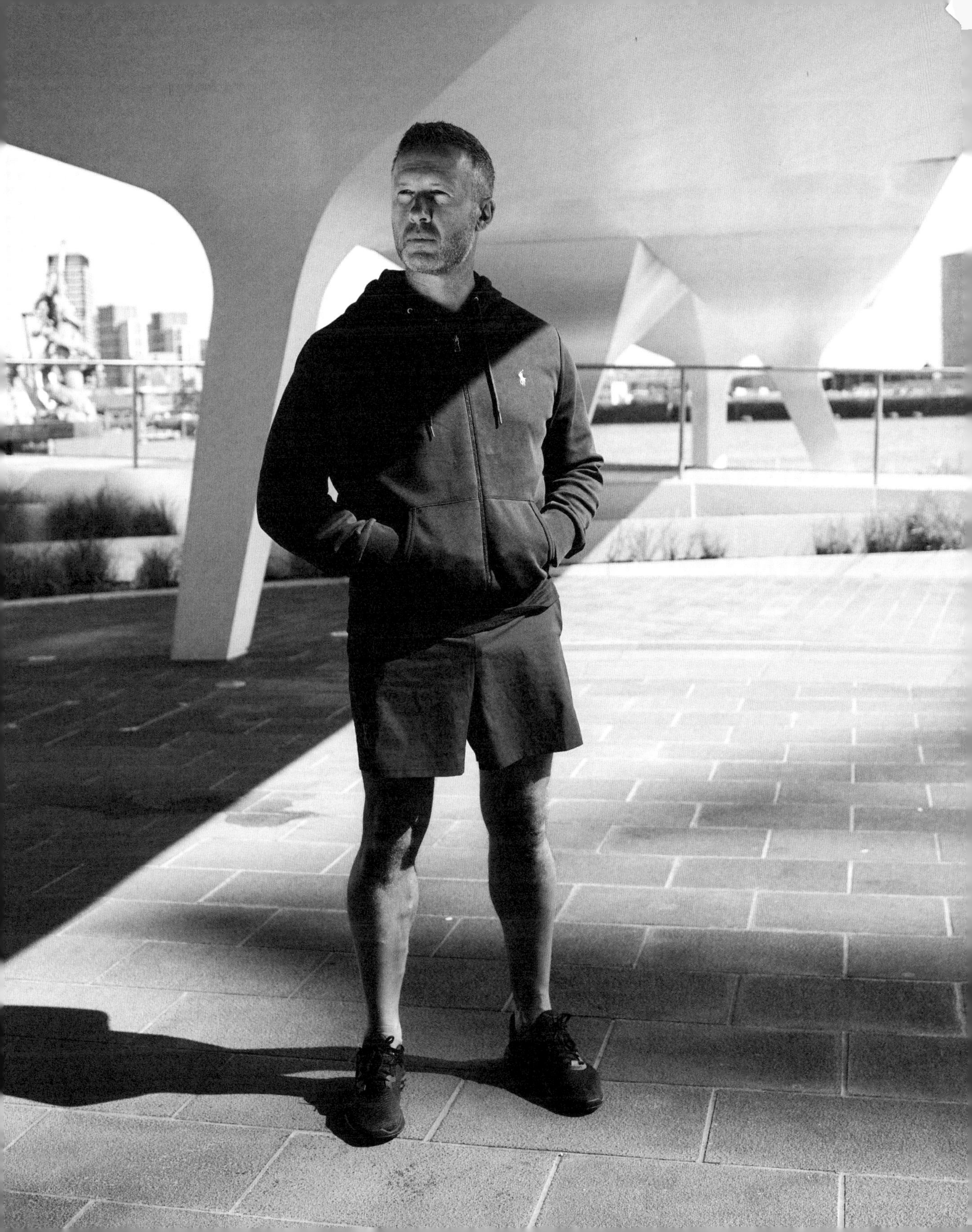

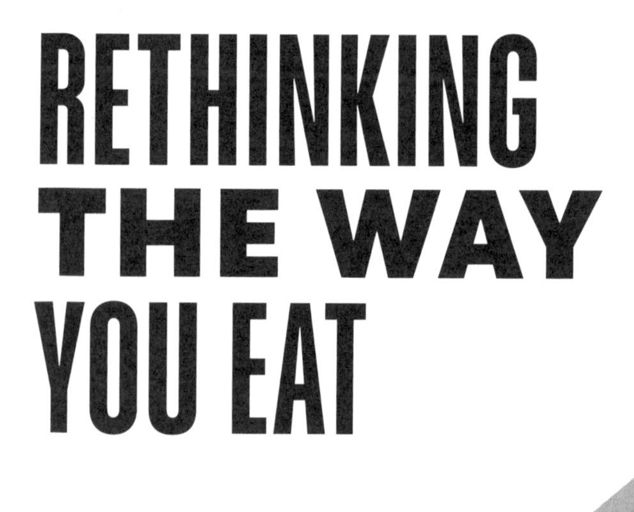

RETHINKING THE WAY YOU EAT

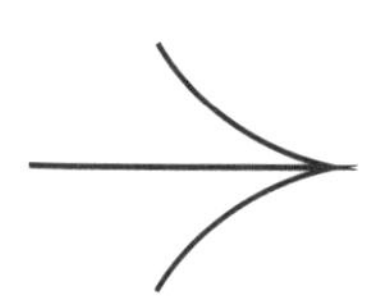

The Six Pack Revolution is designed to make you completely rethink your daily eating habits, which is crucial in today's food culture of ultra-processed, fast food. Unlike many extreme diets, we don't cut out entire food groups. Our recipes are balanced, adaptable, quick to prepare, and bursting with flavour.

EVERYDAY CHANGES FOR LASTING RESULTS

REDEFINING HEALTHY EATING

The Six Pack Revolution advocates for balanced meals that effectively fuel your body. Unlike restrictive diets, our approach doesn't eliminate entire food groups but instead seeks harmony on your plate.

EMBRACE FOOD FREEDOM

With a high-protein diet, the focus shifts to giving your body more of what it needs, not less of what it craves. Experience food freedom with maximum flexibility and no compromise on taste or enjoyment.

CATERING TO YOUR NEEDS

Whether you have food intolerances, allergies, follow a vegan lifestyle, or simply want to try something different, our 'like-for-like' section on pp.24–29 allows everyone to enjoy these flavoursome recipes regardless of their dietary preferences. This feature makes the programme adaptable for everyone by providing easy swaps to suit your needs.

QUICK AND CONVENIENT

In today's busy world, quick solutions are essential. Our recipes can be prepared in 30 minutes or less. Enjoy balanced high-protein meals without sacrificing time or taste.

ELEVATE YOUR PLATE

Experience the full spectrum of taste and nutrition with our high-protein recipes. Infused with flavoursome, health-boosting heroes like ginger, garlic, and cumin, each dish offers a delicious boost of micronutrients, polyphenols, and antioxidants. Say goodbye to bland meals and hello to vibrant, nourishing flavours.

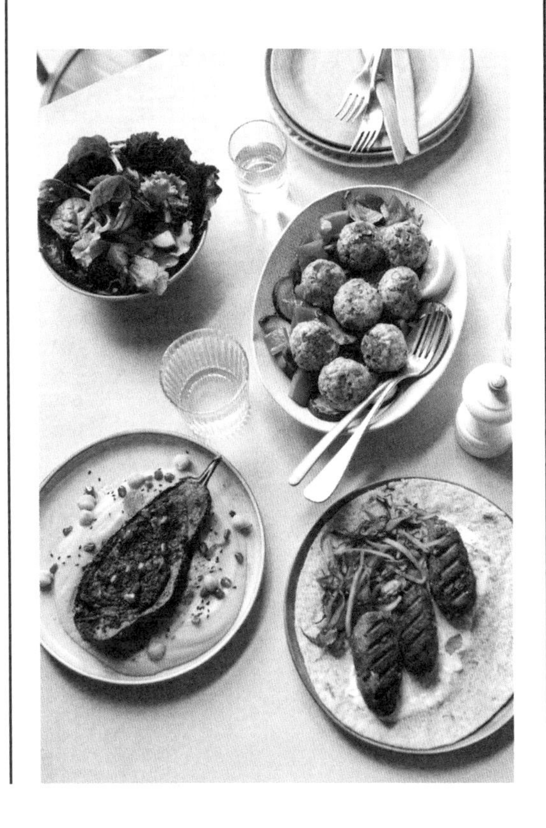

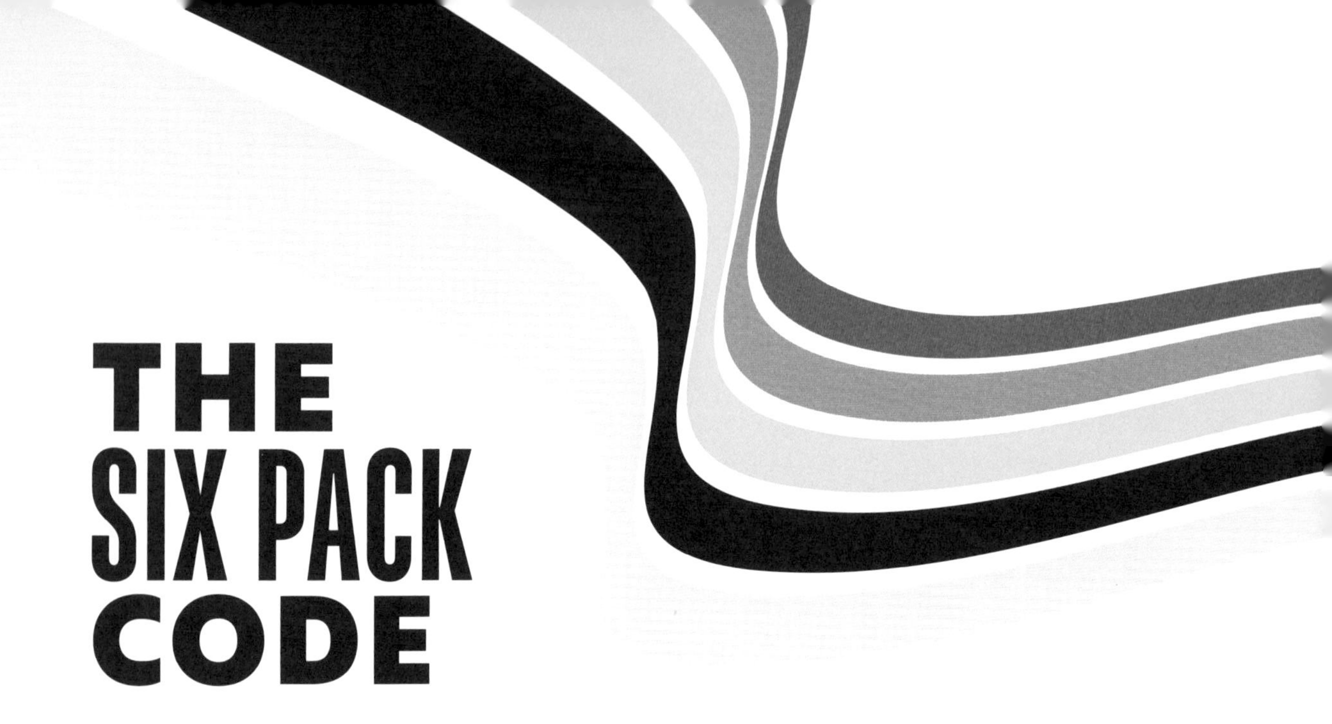

THE SIX PACK CODE

The "Six Pack Code" revolves around THREE pivotal elements:

SIX | RULES | BALANCE

- **SIX – EMBRACE THE POWER OF SIX**
  At the core of The Six Pack Revolution (SPR) lies the principle of eating six times per day – three delicious meals and three satisfying snacks. Enjoy them in any order throughout the day, trying to leave at least 2 hours but no more than 4 hours between eating. Don't add anything or skip any meals or snacks.

- **RULES – THE HAND-PORTION METHOD**
  The science-backed approach of portioning macronutrients is most easily achieved using your hand as a guide.

- **BALANCE – SPR IS ALL ABOUT BALANCE**
  Fuelling your body correctly SIX times a day, using our RULES of the hand creates BALANCE. A balanced plate of food = balanced hormones = peak performance.

THE BENEFITS OF EATING SIX TIMES A DAY

BOOSTING METABOLISM

Fuel your body's furnace by igniting the thermic effect of food (TEF) through frequent eating. Each meal sparks the metabolism, ensuring a steady burn of calories throughout the day.

REGULATING BLOOD SUGAR LEVELS

Say goodbye to energy slumps and cravings with consistent blood sugar levels maintained through regular eating.

ENHANCING FAT BURNING

Keep the flames of fat burning ablaze by providing your body with a continuous stream of nutrients. Optimal nutrient delivery and insulin response foster efficient fat metabolism, aiding in your journey towards a leaner physique.

INCREASING SATIETY

Experience prolonged feelings of fullness and satisfaction throughout the day, curbing the urge to indulge in unhealthy snacking. Embrace a newfound sense of control over your cravings.

LEARNING PORTION CONTROL

Eating six smaller meals/snacks per day prevents binge eating and establishes a habit of portion control for effective weight management.

IMPROVING NUTRIENT DISTRIBUTION

Ensure a balanced intake of essential nutrients by spreading your meals and snacks evenly throughout the day. Empower your body with the fuel it needs to thrive, moment by moment.

STABILIZING MOOD AND MENTAL CLARITY

Say hello to sustained energy levels and heightened cognitive function, courtesy of frequent eating. Maintain focus, productivity, and emotional wellbeing with a steady supply of nourishment.

IMPROVING DIGESTION AND GUT HEALTH

Ease the burden on your digestive system with smaller, more frequent meals/snacks. Embrace improved gut health as you promote smoother digestion and absorption of nutrients.

BALANCING HORMONAL RESPONSE

Nurture hormonal harmony with regular, balanced eating patterns. Support optimal hormone secretion, including those vital for appetite regulation, metabolism, and stress management.

SIMPLE RULE OF THE HAND

You may already be familiar with the rule of the hand, which is a key factor in The Six Pack Revolution. By using your hand as a measuring tool, you can tailor the size of your meals to your unique body dimensions. Using this rule, every plate is customized to meet your individual nutritional needs.

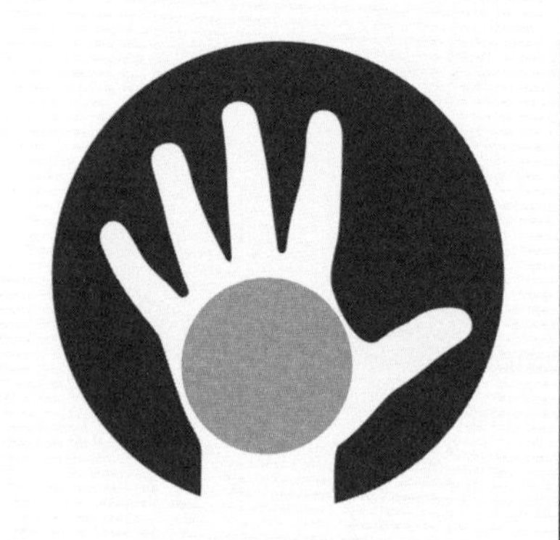

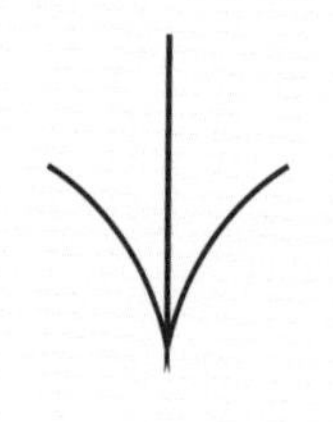

PROTEIN

The size and thickness of your palm

For plant-based protein, aim for 1.5x your palm's size and thickness.

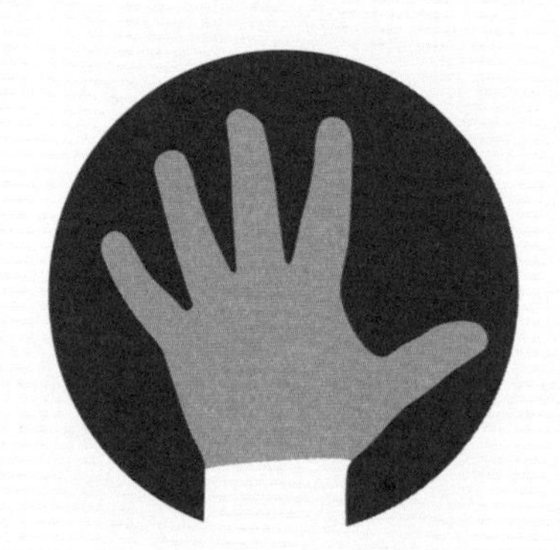

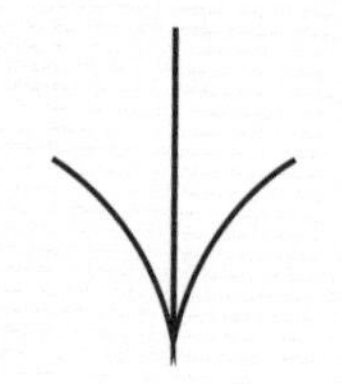

CARBS

Handfuls of goodness

Use the size of your palm and outstretched fingers to guide carb intake per meal.

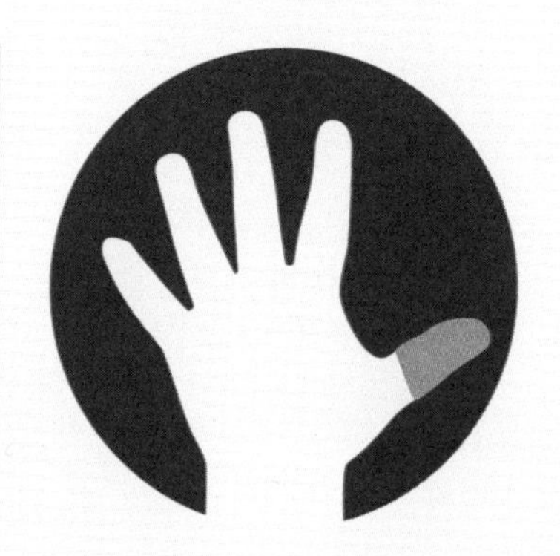

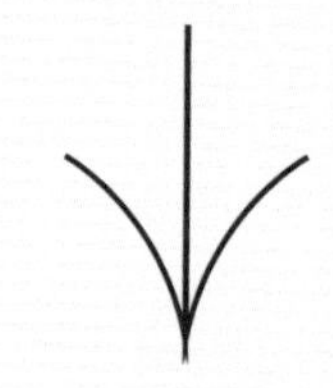

FAT

Just a dash

Use roughly a thumb-sized amount, or as specified in the recipe.

A BALANCING ACT

THE ESSENCE OF THE SIX PACK REVOLUTION

At the heart of The Six Pack Revolution pulses a playful mantra: balance – much like the delicate dance of Yin and Yang, positive and negative, balance permeates every aspect of our lives and serves as the cornerstone of vibrant health, syncing our hormones – which serve as messengers governing an array of physiological functions.

BALANCED HORMONES = PEAK PERFORMANCE

Our team of nutritionists have worked hard to ensure that when fuelling your body the SPR way, you will optimize your metabolism and help balance your body and hormones. Many of our participants have experienced improvements to their body so it works at its optimum, burning unhealthy fat more efficiently, building and maintaining muscle mass, and improving hair, skin, teeth and nails.

You may also find that chronic illnesses become more manageable or brought into remission – we have so much wonderful experience of this when participants follow our programme. A range of health conditions may be completely eradicated or reduced. These include menopausal problems, high blood pressure, increased cholesterol levels, type 1 and 2 diabetes, IBS, Crohns, eczema, psoriasis, arthritis, thyroid function/ Hashimoto's, ME/fibromyalgia, MS, sleep apnoea, scoliosis, lipodema, and Guillain-barré Syndrome (GBS), just to name a few.

LET'S EXPLORE SOME KEY COMPONENTS THAT CONTRIBUTE TO HORMONAL BALANCE

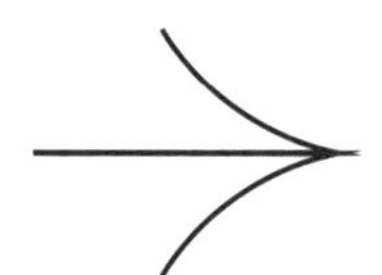

1. PROTEIN: BUILDING BLOCKS OF HEALTH

Protein, the cornerstone of tissue repair and neurotransmitter synthesis, plays a pivotal role in hormonal regulation by providing amino acids. These are the building blocks for neurotransmitters like dopamine, for example, essential for various functions in the brain, including regulating mood, motivation, movement and cognitive function.

> **Good to Know: Key Foods for Boosting Dopamine**
> *Incorporating protein-rich foods into your diet can help boost dopamine levels, enhancing mood and promoting emotional well-being. Opt for lean protein sources such as chicken, turkey, white fish, eggs and tofu to support optimal dopamine production.*

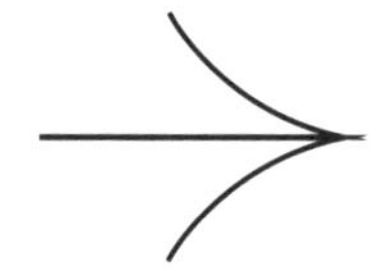

2. THE STRESS RESPONSE: STABILITY INSIGHTS

Ongoing research into our body's stress response continues to shed light on the critical role of diet in stabilizing hormonal fluctuations, including cortisol and adrenaline. Data highlights the stabilizing effect of complex carbohydrates on blood sugar levels, offering a scientific basis for their role in mitigating stress hormone surges.

> **Good to Know: Stress-Relieving Foods**
> *The recipes we create are rich in complex carbohydrates like whole grains, sweet potato, fruits, and vegetables. These ingredients not only aid weight loss when included within a balanced diet but also support stable energy levels and emotional wellbeing. Feedback from participants often includes feelings of calmness and happiness, showcasing the holistic benefits of our approach.*

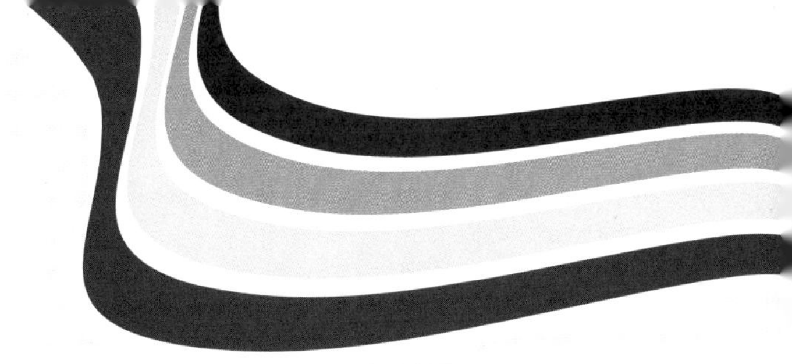

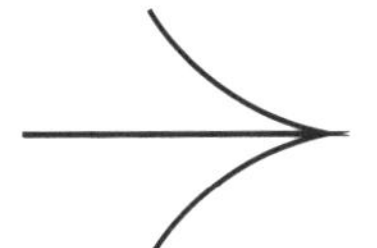

3.OMEGA-3 FATTY ACIDS: PERFECT BRAIN BOOSTERS

In the realm of brain health, data-driven research underscores the significance of omega-3 fatty acids. Studies demonstrate their role in neurotransmitter production, with robust evidence linking their consumption to improved mood regulation and cognitive function.

Good to Know: Sources of Omega-3 Fatty Acids
Incorporating omega-3 fatty acids into your diet can be achieved through consuming fish such as salmon, mackerel and sardines, as well as plant-based sources like olive oil, avocado, nuts, and seeds.

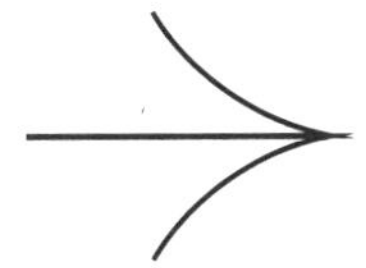

4. ANTIOXIDANTS: HORMONE HEROES

Antioxidants are like superheroes for your hormones – they help keep your hormonal balance in check by fighting off harmful free radicals and reducing oxidative stress. Including antioxidant-rich foods in your diet is key to supporting your hormones and overall well-being.

Good to Know: Foods Packed with Antioxidants
Load up on colourful foods like berries, leafy greens, carrots, bell peppers, and tomatoes. Nuts, seeds, and green tea are also a great source of antioxidants.

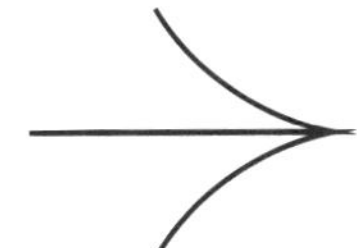

5. HYDRATION: THE FOUNDATION OF CELLULAR HEALTH

Ever wonder why staying hydrated is so important? Hydration isn't just about quenching your thirst—it's a key player in keeping your hormones in check. Adequate water intake helps transport nutrients, detoxifies pathways, and keeps hormone levels in balance, fighting fatigue and increasing energy levels, are all super important.

Good to Know: Recommended Daily Intake
For optimal health, experts recommend women consume around 3 litres (5¼ pints) of water per day, while men are advised to aim for about 4 litres (7 pints).

WHAT WE KNOW . . .
PROTEIN

WHAT ARE PROTEINS?

Proteins are the essential architects of life, crucial for building and repairing muscle tissue, bolstering immune function, and fostering feelings of fullness after eating. Comprised of amino acids, these tiny powerhouses are fundamental to our physiological framework.

Without proteins, our bodies would lack the structural integrity to combat infections, regulate appetite, or conduct basic cellular functions. From supporting muscle growth and repair to orchestrating immune responses, proteins serve as the cornerstone of our health and vitality.

With over 10,000 diverse proteins sculpting and sustaining our essence, it's clear they play a starring role in our nutritional narrative. However, it's essential to exercise caution. Consuming an imbalanced, high-protein diet can put strain on vital organs like the kidneys and liver, disrupting our delicate internal harmony.

Moreover, proteins also play a crucial role in maintaining bone health. Collagen, a protein found abundantly in bone tissue, provides strength and structure to our skeletal system. By ensuring an adequate intake of protein-rich foods, we not only support muscle growth and immune function but also contribute to the maintenance of strong and resilient bones.

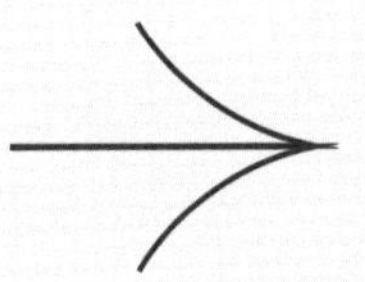

PROTEIN: THE GOOD, THE BAD, AND THE UGLY

- **THE GOOD**
  Whole proteins are nutritional dynamos, offering a wealth of nutrients to fuel your body. From lean meats, like chicken and turkey, to nutrient-dense fish, like white fish, salmon and tuna, these options pack a punch in both taste and nutrition. Plant-based sources like tofu, Quorn and lentils provide ample protein along with fibre and essential vitamins and minerals, making them ideal choices for those seeking a meat-free diet.

- **THE BAD**
  Processed meats come with a host of health concerns. Deli meats, sausages, and bacon are often laden with preservatives, sodium, and unhealthy fats, increasing the risk of heart disease, cancer, and other chronic conditions. Consuming these foods in excess can wreak havoc on your health, so it's best to limit your intake and opt for leaner options like ostrich, or whole, unprocessed alternatives whenever possible. Remember, just because it says "vegan" on the packet doesn't mean it's healthy, in fact, most of the time it's the complete opposite.

- **THE UGLY**
  The rise of protein-centric marketing has given way to a flood of packaged foods promising protein benefits while sacrificing nutritional integrity. These processed imposters masquerading as healthy microwave meals, for example, often contain elevated levels of added sugars, artificial flavours, and preservatives, negating many potential health benefits they may offer. While convenient, these products can sabotage your efforts to maintain a balanced diet and may contribute to weight gain and other health issues over time. So, make sure you choose cleaner, healthier products when looking for a convenient alternative for on-the-go, they do exist.

TAKING THE FOCUS OFF CALORIE COUNTING!

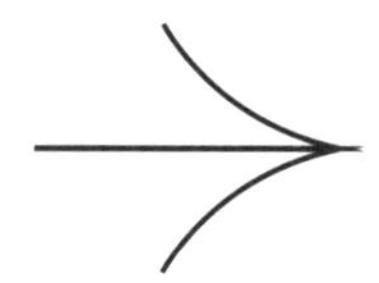

You will notice that in this book and The Six Pack Revolution programme itself we do not focus on calories.

This is intentional and important! People will often tell you that as long as you are in a calorie deficit that's all you need to create for fat loss. Well, this is not the case. Focusing solely on calorie counting can sometimes lead to an overly simplistic approach to weight loss and may not promote overall health. Here are a few reasons why it's beneficial to consider more than just calories when trying to lose fat.

Not all calories are created equal. Foods vary in their nutrient composition, and focusing only on calories can lead to neglecting important nutrients your body needs for optimal health. For example, if you starve yourself all day so you can have some fast food, a pint of fizz and a bag of chocolates in the evening to keep within your calories, this will not work! Prioritizing nutrient-dense foods ensures you're getting essential vitamins, minerals, and other micronutrients necessary for optimum health. Different foods can have varying effects on hunger, satiety levels, and blood sugars, even if they contain the same number of calories. For example, foods high in fibre, protein, and healthy fats tend to be more filling and can help control appetite, maintain blood sugars, give you energy and aid weight loss, making it easier to stick to a healthier diet without feeling deprived.

Rigid calorie counting can be unsustainable for many people and may lead to disordered eating behaviours or an unhealthy relationship with food. Instead, focusing on building healthy, balanced eating habits can promote long-term success. This is much healthier, results are quicker and it is more effective for fat loss when you think about food in a healthy way, rather than trying to drastically cut calories.

INFLAMMATION

It's important to understand why we prioritize removing unnecessary sugar and added salt. Diets high in salt and sugar can lead to inflammation in the body. I've received numerous insightful testimonials from participants, highlighting how the programme has helped them combat various ailments associated with inflammation.

UNDERSTANDING INFLAMMATION IN THE BODY:

Inflammation, a cornerstone of the body's immune response, serves as a double-edged sword. While acute inflammation is a vital defence mechanism against pathogens and injury, chronic inflammation poses a significant threat to our wellbeing. Persistent, low-grade inflammation, often fuelled by dietary and lifestyle factors, can lead to a host of health complications, including cardiovascular disease, diabetes, autoimmune disorders and even cancer. Every cell in your body is nourished or malnourished based on what we eat and drink.

THE ROLE OF DIET IN INFLAMMATION:

The gut, often referred to as the "second brain", plays a crucial part in regulating inflammatory processes. Consuming processed and refined foods laden with excess salt, sugar and sweeteners disrupts the delicate balance of the gut microbiome, paving the way for systemic inflammation.

By simply minimizing our sugar and salt intake consuming only natural salts and sugars found within healthy unprocessed foods, we can reduce the risk of chronic diseases like diabetes, heart disease, fatty liver disease, certain cancers and many more.

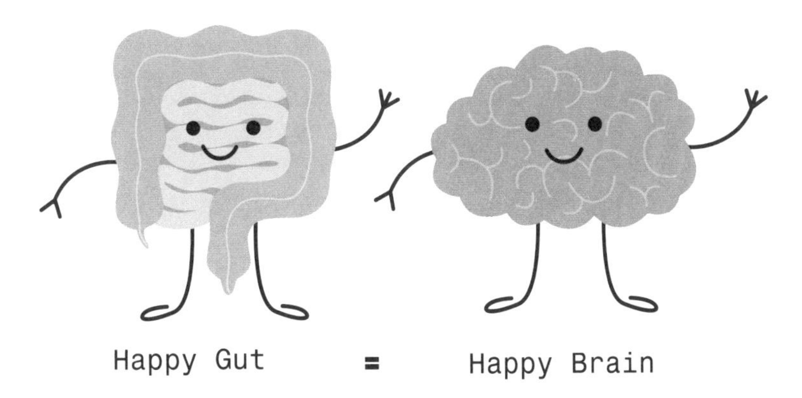

Happy Gut = Happy Brain

LIKE-FOR-LIKE SWAPS

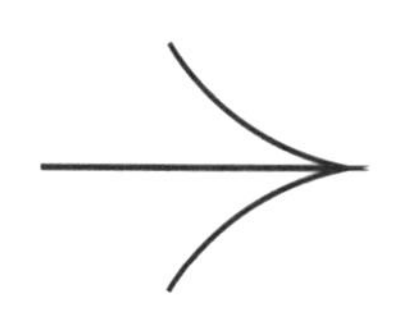

ELEVATING FLAVOUR, EMBRACING VARIETY

You're nearly ready to cook up a treat with our delicious and speedy high-protein recipes. Within each recipe, there is plenty of flexibility to accommodate various dietary preferences. Each dish is thoughtfully curated to ensure that every ingredient swap, whether it be for non-dairy or meat-free alternatives, enhances the richness and depth of flavour, promising a balanced dining experience that is equally delicious and satisfying for all palates.

Take a look at pages 26–29 for my swap guidelines.

PLANT PROTEIN SWAPS: THE ESSENTIALS

Swapping meat for plant-based proteins can be a delightful culinary adventure with a host of health benefits. Here's everything you need to make the best choices.

- **Tofu:** Made from soyabeans (soybeans), comes in firm or silken. Firm tofu is best for stir-fries, grilling, and baking while silken tofu is ideal for smoothies, desserts, and soups.
- **Tempeh:** A fermented soya (soy) product with a firm texture, perfect for frying, grilling, or crumbling into dishes.
- **Seitan:** Made from wheat gluten, seitan has a chewy texture and works well in dishes in place of meat and fish.
- **Quorn:** A mycoprotein that mimics the texture of meat and is excellent for chilli, curry, and stews.
- **Vegan Chicken:** Plant-based chicken alternatives can be used in place of traditional chicken or turkey in most recipes (make sure they are unflavoured).

UNLOCKING THE BENEFITS OF EATING LEGUMES

Do not over consume foods like chickpeas, beans, and lentils as they can be stodgy, hard to digest, and cause bloating. They also contain lectins and phytates, which when eaten too often can cause leaky gut. Stick to once or twice a week and you'll be fine.

CAN YOU REPLACE ANY PROTEIN WITH ANY OTHER?

While you can generally swap plant proteins for meat in most of my recipes, do consider the texture and flavour profile of the substitute.

- **Chicken:** Use tempeh, seitan, or vegan chicken for a similar texture. Firm tofu or Quorn pieces or strips can also be great substitutes.
- **Minced (Ground) Meat:** Try lentils, crumbled tofu or tempeh, and Quorn (Grounds) or soya mince (soy crumbles).
- **Fish:** Firm tofu or Quorn are great substitutes as they can mimic the texture of "meaty" fish.

THE BENEFITS OF LEGUMES

From ancient diets to modern plates, legumes have been a dietary staple for centuries, offering many health benefits. Here are all the reasons why these small wonders are used so frequently in my recipes...

- **Chickpeas:** Rich in folate, vitamin B6, and vitamin C, chickpeas bolster immune function and support heart health. Folate aids cell growth, vitamin B6 enhances cognitive function, and vitamin C boosts collagen production for vibrant skin.
- **Beans:** Packed with folate, thiamine, and niacin, beans fuel energy metabolism and nerve function. They also provide minerals, like iron and magnesium, for blood oxygenation and muscle function.
- **Lentils:** High in folate, iron, and potassium, lentils promote blood health, nerve function, and fluid balance. Folate supports DNA synthesis, iron boosts energy production, and potassium regulates blood pressure.

LET'S EXPLORE HOW TO SWAP KEY MACROS IN YOUR DIET

PROTEIN KINGS

SPR PROTEINS	HOW TO SWAP	MEAT-FREE PROTEINS	GOOD TO KNOW
Meat/Fish Proteins Chicken Mussels Ostrich Prawns Rabbit Salmon Tuna Steak Tinned tuna in spring water Turkey White fish	A palm-size and thickness of meat protein is equivalent to:	Alternative protein sources should be basic plain soya (soy) chunks or tofu, tempeh, soya or seitan with no extra flavourings. *Please note if you are considering using other vegan protein options, they must be < 5g fat and approx. 1g salt per 100g (3½oz).*	Avoid prepared/deli style meat and anything that is flavoured or formed into a burger, sausage or fried food.
Vegetarian/Vegan Proteins Quorn Tofu Seitan Soya mince (soy crumbles) Tempeh Vegan chicken	1.5 palm-size and thickness of vegetarian/vegan protein.		
Legumes Chickpeas Beans (various) Lentils	1x 400g (14oz) can of legumes, drained and rinsed, OR 100g (3½oz) of dry legumes.		

VEGGIE POWER HOUSES

VEGGIES OF CHOICE	HOW TO SWAP	SKIP THE STARCH	GOOD TO KNOW
These are my favourites: Aubergine (eggplant) Asparagus Broccoli Brussels sprouts Carrots Courgette (zucchini) Green beans Kale Mixed leaf salad Peppers Peas Parsnip Spinach Swede(rutabaga) Sweetcorn Sweet potato	Switch any veggie goodness with your favourite colourful veg… remember, an outstretched handful is your measure.	The only vegetable (tuber) that doesn't appear in our recipes is the white potato. This is not because they are bad, it's just that sweet potatoes are far more nutritious with a high level of antioxidants and a low glycemic index, which is great for managing blood sugars.	Do not swap vegetables for fruit. These delicious veggies are not for snacking. Only use as part of one of our recipes.

SMART CARBS

CARBOHYDRATES	HOW TO SWAP	DRY VS COOKED	GOOD TO KNOW
Bulgur wheat Buckwheat Freekah Plain couscous Quinoa *These carbs are measured by weight and not by the hand portion method.*	Not feeling your couscous tonight? You can swap it out for another smart carb. If following a recipe, remember to follow the portion size of that ingredient when swapping as each recipe will differ.	Rule of thumb on grains... The dry weight equals 2.5–3 times the weight when cooked. For example, if the recipe states 150g (5½oz) of cooked quinoa, you will only need 50g (1¾oz) of the dry weight.	These smart carbs are just that – they support heart health, aid digestion with their high-fibre content, and provide essential nutrients for overall wellbeing.

OUR FIRM FRUITY FAVOURITES

FRUITILICIOUS	HOW TO SWAP	OTHER FRUITS	GOOD TO KNOW
Apple Banana Blackberries Blueberries Cherries Kiwi Mango Melon Nectarine Papaya Peach Pineapple Raspberries Strawberries Watermelon	Feeling berry-less? Swap them out for another fruit, just remember to stick to the portion in the recipe.	We are all about flavour, so if you have a fruit that you love, be sure to try it out in any of our meals or snacks that contain fruit.	Although it's tempting to grab a banana on the go, remember balance is key so choose a healthy SPR recipe instead.

GOOD FATS GALORE

HEALTHY FATS	FOR COOKING	FOR SALADS	GOOD TO KNOW
Unsalted nuts 6 almonds 6 cashews 6 hazelnuts 6 pecan halves 8 pistachios 6 walnut halves 2 teaspoons of desiccated coconut OR mixed seeds (*chia, pumpkin, sunflower, sesame, flax, hemp*) 6 olives ½ avocado	**Teaspoon of...** Coconut oil Extra virgin olive oil Rapeseed (Canola) oil Sesame oil	Include ½ avocado as a swap for oil in salads. They are nutrient dense and rich in healthy fats, which support heart health. They are also high in fibre, aiding digestion and promoting satiety, and a good source of vitamins as well as folate, magnesium, and potassium.	Don't skip healthy fats. They are essential for brain function, hormone production and overall cell health.

HYDRATION HEROES

WATER	JAZZ IT UP	OTHER BEVERAGES	GOOD TO KNOW
For optimal health, experts recommend women drink around 3 litres (5¼ pints) of water per day, while men are advised to aim for about 4 litres (7 pints).	Tired of plain water? Elevate it with a refreshing twist of fresh lemon, lime or mint for a burst of flavour. Avoid shop-bought infusions and added sugars like honey.	Indulge in up to 2 cups of black, unsweetened caffeinated coffee or tea per day, while savouring unlimited caffeine-free tea.	Craft your own tea by steeping fresh herbs, ginger, mint, cucumber, or lemon in hot water for an infusion that is both refreshing and invigorating.

DAIRY-FREE DELIGHTS

YOGURT ALTERNATIVES	MILK ALTERNATIVES	OTHER OPTIONS	GOOD TO KNOW
We love Greek yogurt but there are alternatives. Replace with sugar free Greek-style soya (soy) yogurt for sweet or savoury dishes.	When a recipe calls for soya (soy) milk, only pea milk or hemp milk are suitable alternatives. Make sure they are unsweetened. Almond milk does not contain protein and oat milk is too high in carbohydrates.	Lactose-free milk and yogurt alternatives are also widely available from most supermarkets.	Our choice of preference is full-fat. Quite often, products with 0% fat can contain added sugars and preservatives.

PLANNING IT ALL OUT

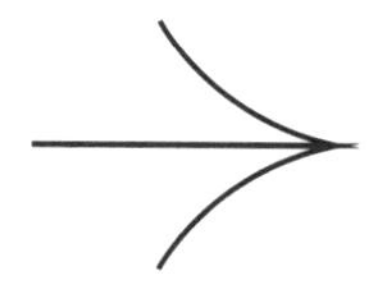

This programme is simple – you choose three meals and three snacks from the recipes in this book, which you can eat in any order throughout the day. However, try and keep a minimum of 2 hours and a maximum of 4 hours between eating, so plan your day accordingly. On the days that you work out only, have a post workout protein smoothie afterwards. This is in addition to the three meals and three snacks.

WHAT IS THE MEAL REPLACEMENT FOOD PLAN?

While you can follow the six pack programme using the recipes that follow in the next few chapters, you can also replace some meals and snacks with meal replacement shakes. Many people who follow this programme have two meals, two snacks, and two meal replacement shakes a day, following each workout with one of our Post Workout Protein Shakes (www.thesixpackrevolution.com/shop). These creamy, delicious Meal Replacement and Post Workout Protein Shakes are made with the highest-quality ingredients. You can also buy our Overnight Oats and Sculpt Protein bars to use as snack options. This typical day is designed to give you an idea of how you might plan your meals. You can use this or download a meal planner and tracker here to make it a little easier.

thesixpackrevolution.com/tracker/

MY DAILY ROUTINE

If you are finding it hard to visualize how to use my *High Protein Meals in Minutes* recipe book then have a look at my perfect day – eating every 2–4 hours, completely on plan and packed with delicious food.

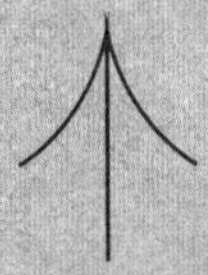

8:00am
SNACK
Smoked Salmon with Sweet Melon and Mint (p.150) OR 1 serving of The Six Pack Revolution meal replacement shake

9:00am
WORKOUT
Try one of my workout challenges (pp.158–208)

10:15am
POST WORKOUT SHAKE
The Six Pack Revolution Decadent Chocolate Caramel Post Workout Protein Shake

11:30am
MEAL
Peking Flatbread with Sweet Chilli Sauce (p.50)

2:00pm
MEAL
Marinated Tofu and Apple Salad (p.60) OR 1 serving of The Six Pack Revolution Meal Replacement Shake

4:00pm
SNACK
Sweet Potato and Banana Pancakes (p.127)

6:30pm
MEAL
Turkey Meatballs and Stir-fry Vegetables (p.118)

9:00pm
SNACK
Raspberry Ripple Smoothie (p.125) OR The Six Pack Revolution Sculpt Bar

MEALS IN MINUTES

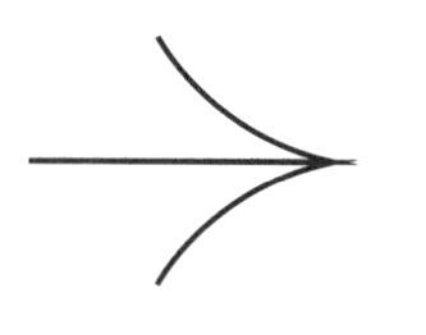

SHOP ONCE. COOK ONCE. EAT WELL ALL WEEK!

If there's one valuable piece of advice I can offer for transforming your eating habits and to save you time in the kitchen, it's this: prioritize preparation. Dedicate time to a single shopping trip and one cooking session.

This straightforward approach saves time and enables you to craft an array of delectable recipes in one go, ensuring you have nutritious meals at the ready all week long. Choose recipes that can be cooked in larger batches and that are effortlessly re-heatable or freezable for maximum convenience.

Many of the recipes in this book will take no longer than 30 minutes to prepare, and some take as little as five minutes! Remember the rules for the meals here: a palm-sized and thickness amount of protein, an outstretched handful of healthy carbohydrates, and your healthy fats!

TIPS FOR COOKING SUCCESS

PLAN YOUR WEEK

Set yourself up for success by planning meals and snacks ahead of time. Preparation is key to staying on track and will save you getting caught short.

LABEL LAWS

Always label containers with the contents and date of freezing to keep track of freshness. Remove them from the freezer the night before to save time the next day.

BATCH-COOKING BRILLIANCE

Spend a couple of hours batch cooking. Freeze or refrigerate extra portions for quick meals during busy times. Your future self will thank you!

SPICY FACTS

When batch cooking, go easy on strong spices like chilli or paprika. Flavours intensify over time, so start small and adjust to your taste.

RECIPE READING ESSENTIALS

Before you dive into cooking, read the entire recipe. Familiarize yourself with the steps and ingredients to avoid surprises that can add time.

ENJOY THE JOURNEY

Cooking is an adventure. Embrace mistakes, enjoy the creative process, and build your skills at your own pace. Nourish your body and find joy in every meal!

PREP LIKE A PRO

Get all your ingredients and equipment ready before you start, then you won't waste time when you could be cooking.

TIMING IS KEY

Many of the recipes in this book are designed to be prepared in 30 minutes or less. Quinola recipes may take a little longer, although if you batch cook these ahead of time you can enjoy them when it suits you.

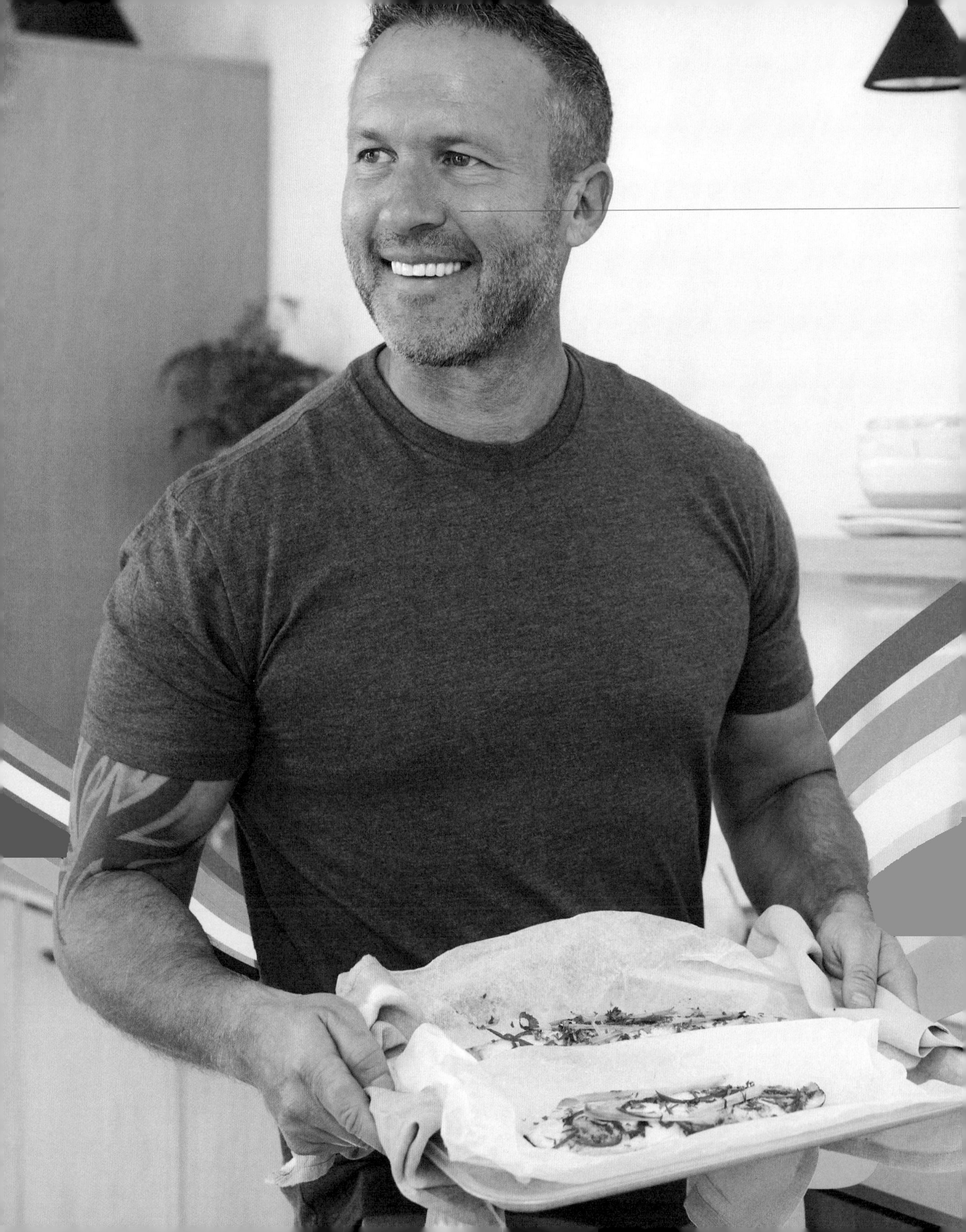

LET'S GET COOKING

Chapter 2

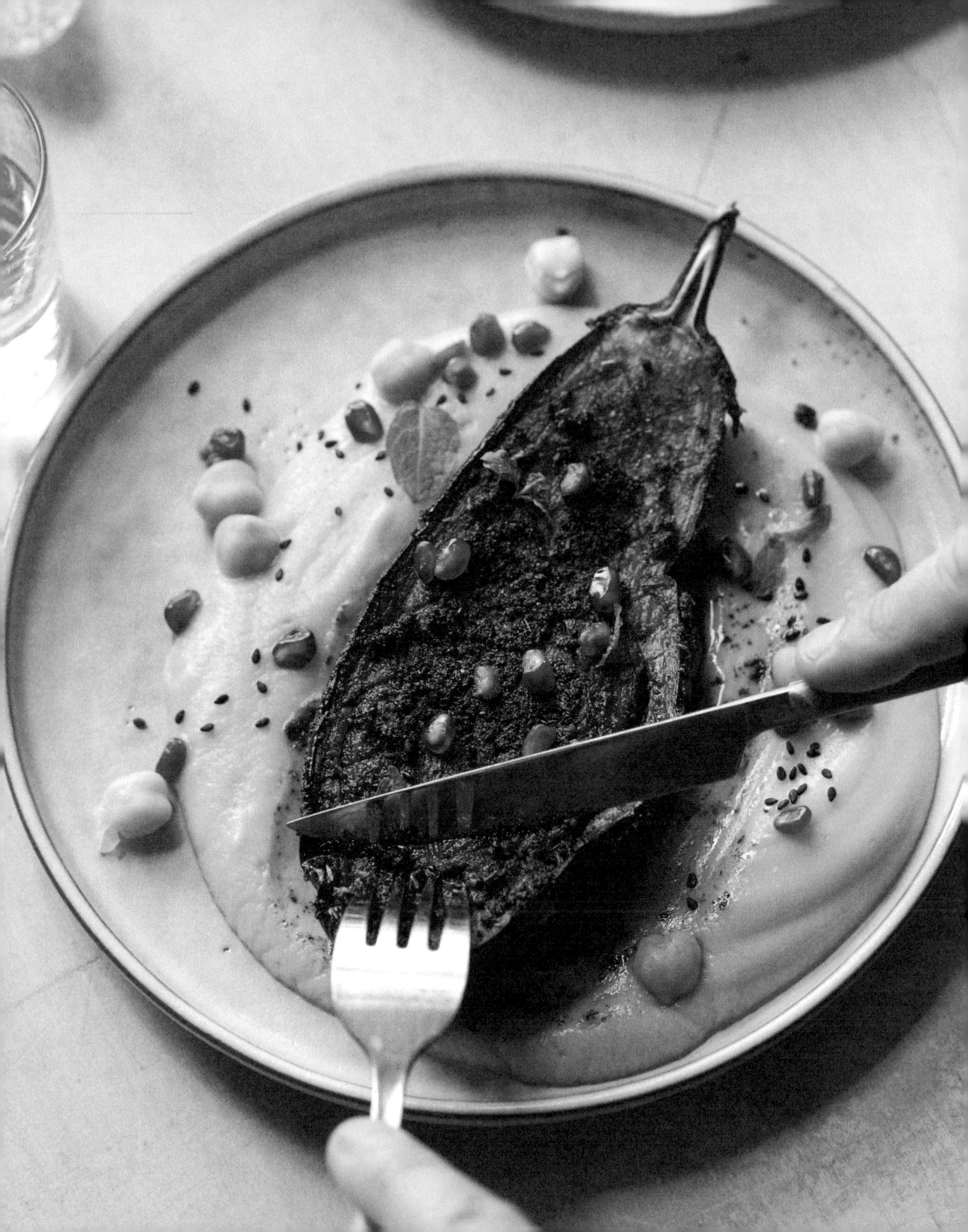

Here is a collection of my most-loved high-protein recipes, created to nourish you every day of your transformation journey. Simply enjoy good food, and you'll start to feel the benefits right away.

MEALS

WHITE BEAN SALAD

SERVES ONE

½ a handful of cooked beetroot (beets), cut into quarters

400g (14oz) can of butter (lima) beans, drained and rinsed

½ orange, peeled and segmented

6 walnuts halves, chopped

watercress leaves to garnish

FOR THE DRESSING

1 tsp fennel seeds

juice and zest of ½ orange

1 tsp dried tarragon

½ tsp ground white pepper

Light, easy, quick, fresh, and tasty! Adding beetroot to your diet can help improve your blood flow, lower blood pressure and increase your exercise performance.

1. Prepare the dressing by lightly toasting the fennel seeds in a non-stick frying pan over a medium heat for 1 minute then transfer to a pestle and mortar and crush.
2. Transfer the crushed seeds to a small mixing bowl then add the remaining dressing ingredients and whisk well.
3. Add the beetroot, butter beans, and salad dressing to a bowl, mix well, and transfer to a salad bowl.
4. Arrange the orange segments around the salad. Sprinkle with the chopped walnuts and garnish with watercress.

FALAFAL BURGER

SERVES ONE

- 400g (14oz) can of chickpeas, drained and rinsed
- handful of fresh flat-leaf parsley and mint
- 1 tsp ras el hanout
- 1 tsp extra virgin olive oil
- 1 combined handful of grated beetroot (beets), apple, and carrot
- freshly ground black pepper

FOR THE TOMATO SALSA

- 1 tomato, diced
- ¼ red onion, diced
- 1 spring (green) onion, sliced
- small handful of fresh, chopped coriander (cilantro)
- 1 tbsp sweetcorn
- juice of ½ lime
- ¼ tsp smoked paprika

This Middle Eastern-inspired meal really shows you what you can do with flavour. Add crunch from the beetroot and carrot with the zing from the tomato salsa, put it all together and boom... street food at its best.

1. Preheat the oven to 180°C (160°C fan/350°F/Gas 4).
2. Prepare the tomato salsa by combining all the ingredients and refrigerate.
3. Place half of the chickpeas in a blender with the parsley, mint, and ras el hanout and blend until smooth (this can be done with a potato masher if you do not have a blender).
4. In a mixing bowl, combine the whole chickpeas and the blended chickpea paste.
5. Form a burger-style patty from the chickpea mixture and put it in the fridge to set for 15 minutes.
6. Place a non-stick frying pan over a medium heat, add the olive oil and pan fry the burger for 2 minutes on each side until golden brown, then transfer to a baking tray and cook in the oven to cook for a further 10 minutes.
7. Arrange the grated salad on a plate, add the burger, dress with the tomato salsa, and season with black pepper.

TUNA AND POMEGRANATE SALAD WITH A RASPBERRY AND HERB DRESSING

SERVES ONE

large combined handful of salad to include: mixed green salad leaves, green beans, spring (green) onion, and courgette (zucchini) ribbons

1 tbsp pomegranate seeds

canned tuna in spring water, the size and thickness of your palm, drained

FOR THE DRESSING

6 raspberries

1 tsp extra virgin olive oil

pinch of dried mixed herbs

pinch of chilli flakes

You may think that tuna with the sweetness of the pomegranate is a strange combination, however, give it a try. This salad is surprisingly tasty and the combination of lean fish, fruit, and vegetables is super healthy.

1. Begin by making the green salad. In a bowl, mix together the green salad leaves, green beans, spring onion, and courgette ribbons. Then add the pomegranate seeds and mix evenly through the salad. Finally, add the tuna, breaking it into large flakes.

2. Now make the dressing. Take the raspberries and mush through a sieve or strainer with the back of a teaspoon, extracting all the juice out of the raspberries, just leaving the pips.

3. Combine the olive oil, mixed herbs, chilli flakes, and raspberry juice in a small dish or jar and stir well.

4. Drizzle the dressing over the tuna salad and serve.

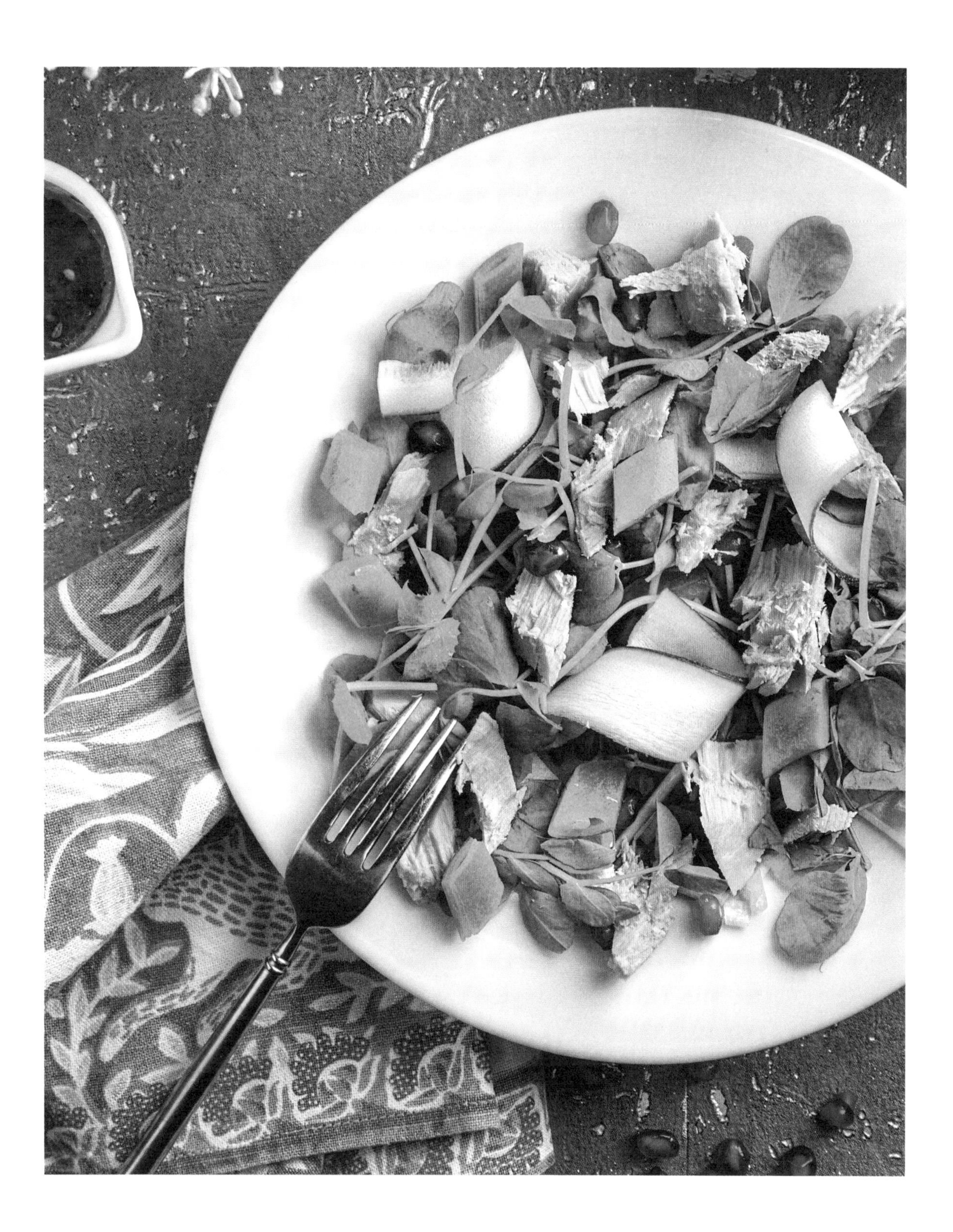

TLT
TOFU LETTUCE TOMATO
SERVES ONE

- ¼ tsp paprika
- ¼ tsp cayenne pepper
- firm tofu, 1½ x the size and thickness of your palm
- 1 tsp full-fat Greek yogurt OR Greek-style soya-based vegan yogurt
- 1 tomato, sliced
- few slices of red onion
- 1–2 Little Gem lettuce leaves
- ½ avocado, sliced
- 1 green olive
- wedge of lemon
- freshly ground black pepper

Raise your lunch game with this protein-packed TLT. Did you know tofu doesn't have its own flavour so easily absorbs any flavour of your choosing? In this recipe, I want our tofu to take on a smoky chilli taste, so I'm coating it with ground cayenne pepper and paprika.

1. Mix the paprika and cayenne pepper together and slice the block of tofu horizontally through the centre to create two flat slices ready to toast.
2. Coat all sides of the tofu with the spices, place them under a medium to high grill (broiler) and toast both sides until turning brown.
3. When the tofu is ready, remove from the grill, and transfer to a plate. Spread the Greek yogurt onto one side of each tofu slice and layer the rest of the ingredients on top of one of the slices to make the filling.
4. Close the sandwich by placing the tofu slice without the filling on top of the other slice. Garnish with an olive and finish with a big squeeze of lemon and some black pepper.

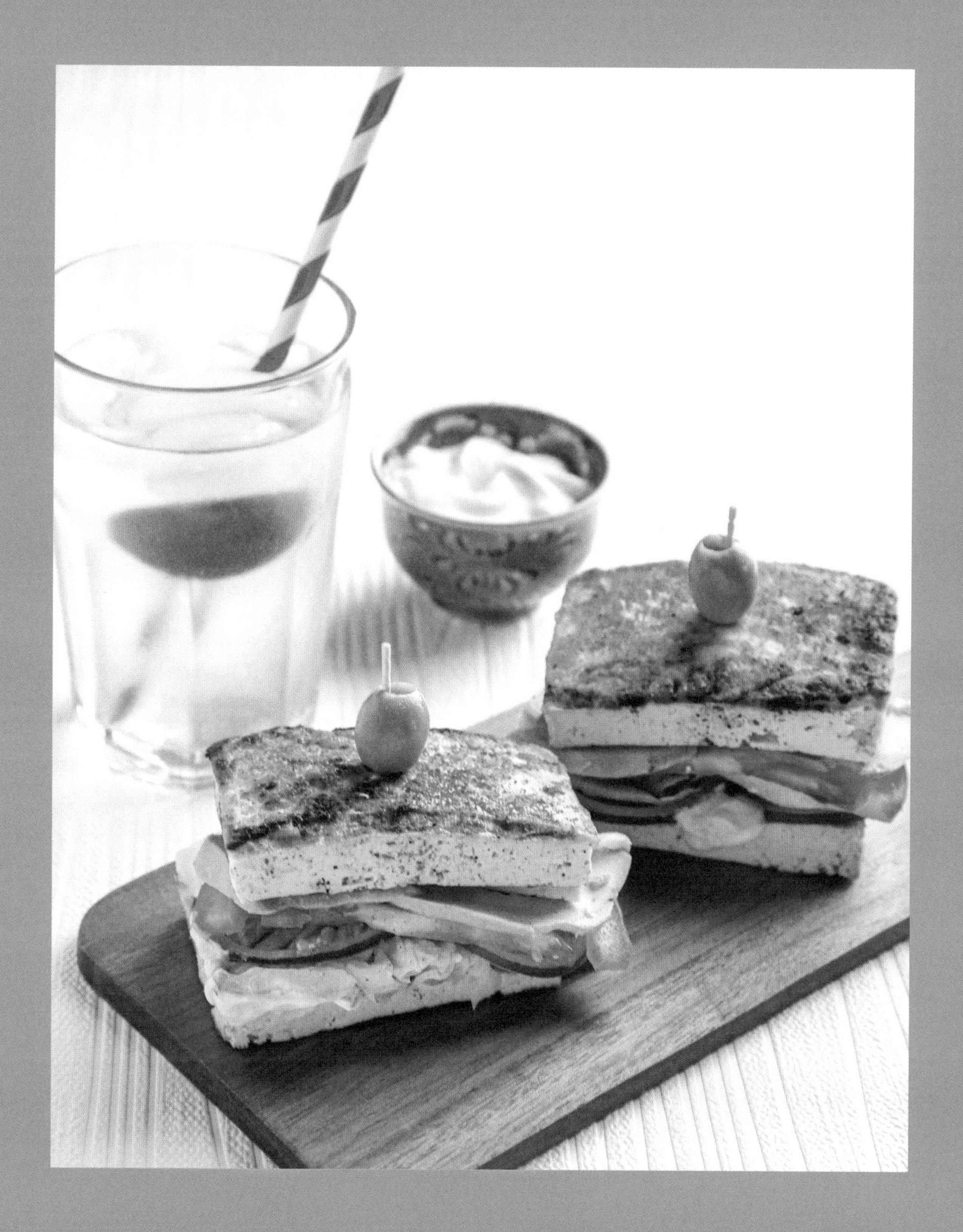

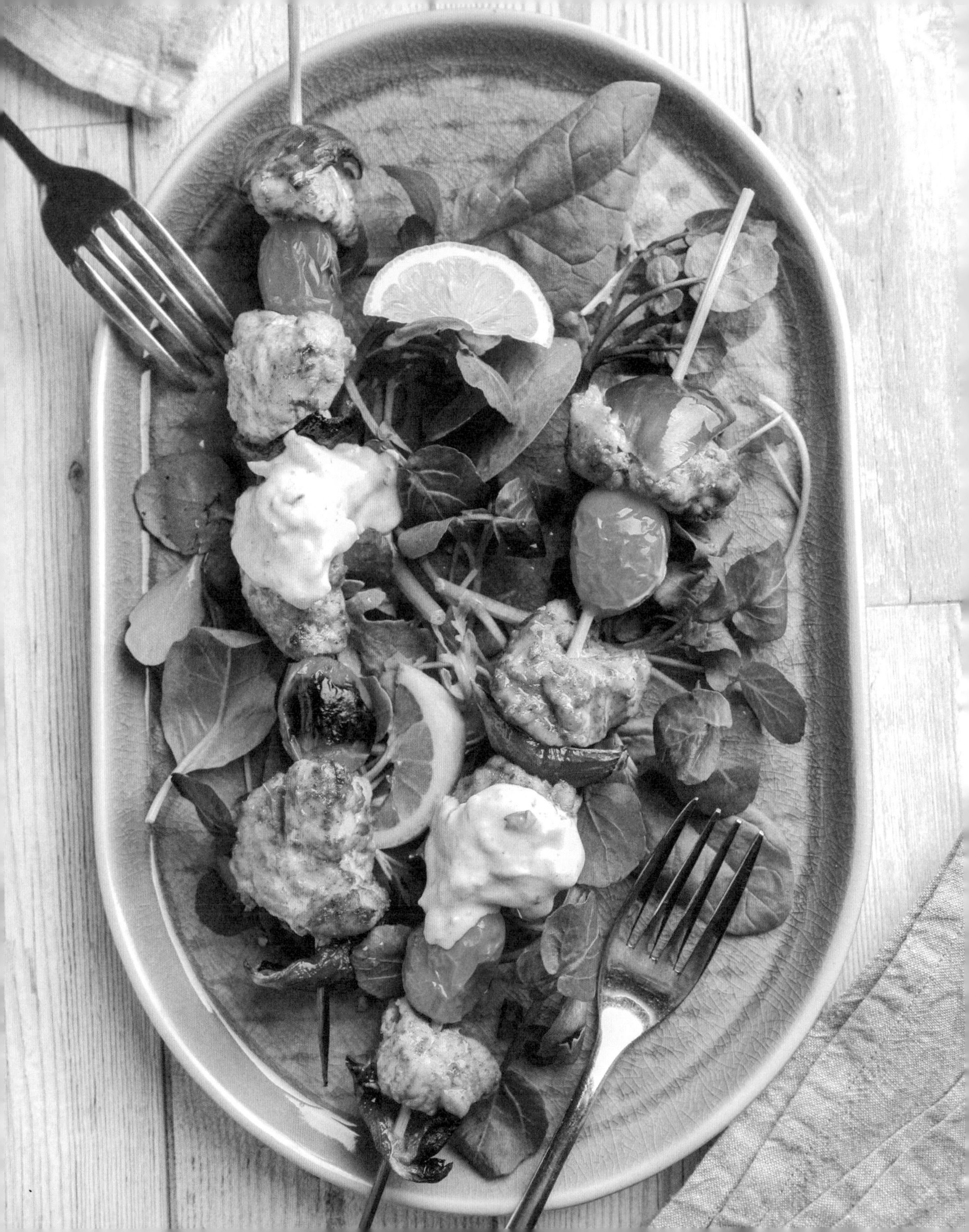

MONKFISH VINDALOO SKEWERS

SERVES TWO

monkfish fillet, 2 x the size and thickness of your palm, cut into large cubes
1 tsp garam masala
¼ tsp hot chilli powder
1 tsp grated fresh ginger root
1 garlic clove, crushed
2 tsp extra virgin olive oil
½ small red onion, cut into big chunks
4 baby plum tomatoes

TO SERVE

handful of mixed salad leaves
1 tbsp raita (optional)
2 lemon wedges

FOR THE RAITA

400g (14oz) full-fat Greek yogurt OR Greek-style soya-based vegan yogurt
½ cucumber, grated and lightly squeezed to remove excess water
½ bunch fresh, chopped coriander (cilantro)
½ bunch fresh, chopped mint
½ tsp garam masala
1–2 garlic cloves, crushed
½ lime, squeezed

Packed full of vitamin B12, and omega-3 fatty acids, monkfish is a stellar choice for boosting heart health and optimal brain function. Its steak-like texture also makes it the ultimate hero to boss your skewers.

1 Coat the cubes of monkfish in the spices, ginger, garlic, and olive oil.

2 Divide the coated monkfish into two equal portions and thread it on to two skewers with the onion and tomatoes. Place under a medium-high grill (broiler) for approximately 15 minutes, turning frequently until the fish is cooked through.

3 Prepare the raita by combining all the ingredients in a bowl.

4 Serve on your favourite plates with a handful of leaves, a tablespoon of raita, if using, and a wedge of lemon.

GOOD TO KNOW

Put the raita in an airtight container and it will last in the fridge for a few days or, alternatively, you can freeze it in a couple of separate freezer bags and it will last a month.

CHINESE SEITAN LETTUCE WRAPS

SERVES TWO

- 1 tsp sesame oil
- seitan slices, 3 x the size and thickness of your palm, chopped into small cubes
- 4 spring (green) onions, finely sliced
- 1 tsp Chinese five spice
- 1 tsp extra virgin olive oil
- 2 closed cup mushrooms, finely chopped
- ½ mango, chopped into small cubes
- 4 Little Gem lettuce leaves
- 1 tbsp fresh, chopped coriander (cilantro)
- 2 wedges of lemon

Seitan is a great alternative to chicken and unlike tofu or tempeh, which are made from soya beans (soybeans). It also has a great texture that combines well with other flavours. This recipe has a solid spice kick and a freshness from the mango and lettuce.

1 Heat the sesame oil in a non-stick frying pan over a medium heat and stir-fry the seitan with the spring onions and half of the five spice for 5 minutes.

2 Add the olive oil and mushrooms and cook for a further 2 minutes. Remove from the heat, add the mango, and stir together.

3 Put two large lettuce leaves on each plate, load them with the seitan mixture, garnish with coriander, and serve with a wedge of lemon.

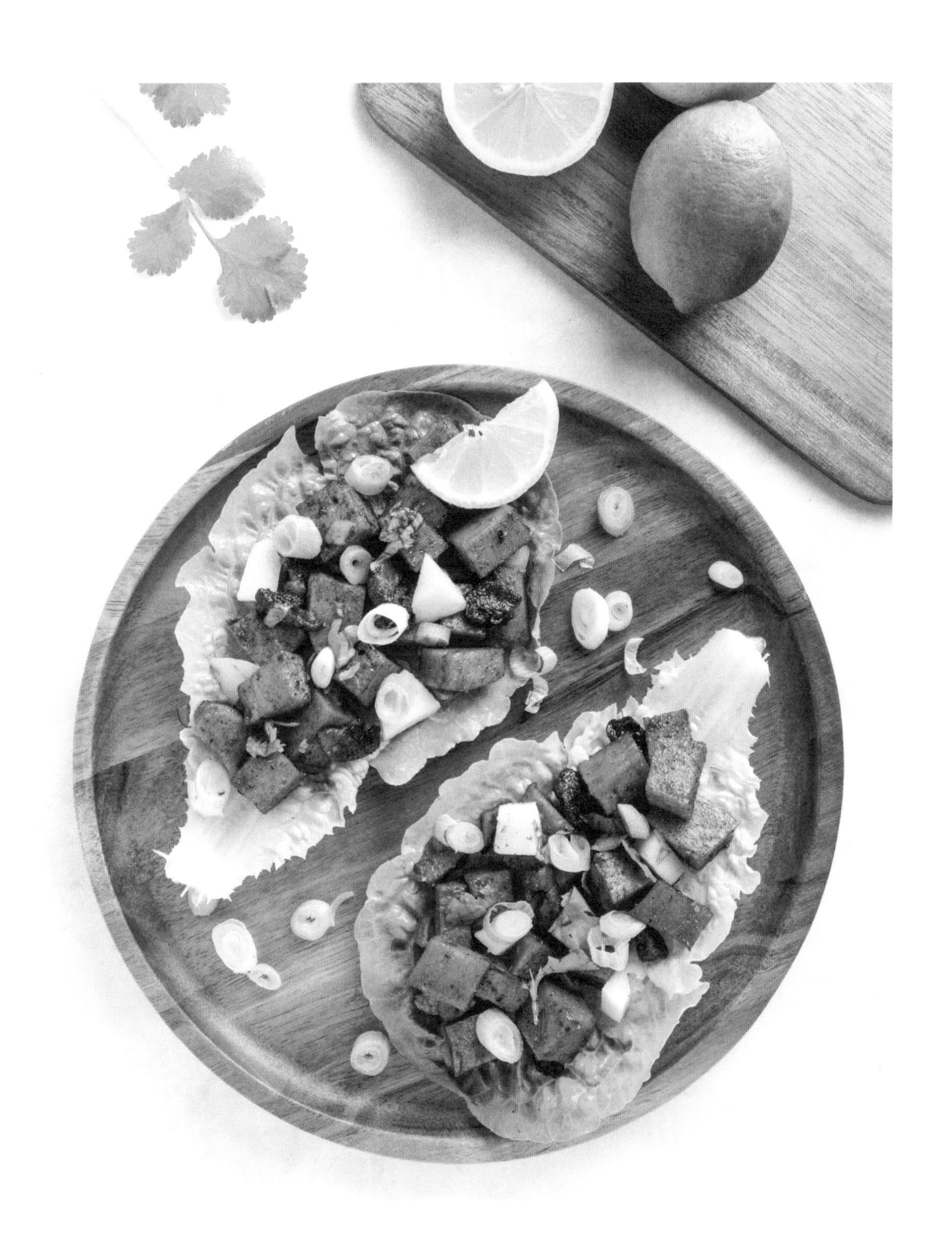

MIXED BEAN CHILLI WITH SWEET POTATO, LIME AND HERBS

SERVES THREE

- handful of sweet potato, peeled and diced
- 1 tsp rapeseed (Canola) oil
- 1 small white onion, finely chopped
- 4 garlic cloves, chopped
- 1 tsp smoked paprika
- 1 tsp mild chilli powder
- 1 tsp ground cumin
- 1 tsp ground coriander
- 2 x 400g (14oz) cans of chopped tomatoes
- large handful of quinoa
- juice and zest of 1 lime
- handful of fresh, chopped coriander (cilantro)
- 3 x 400g (14oz) cans of mixed beans, drained and rinsed
- handful of sweetcorn
- 1 avocado, diced
- large pinch of pumpkin seeds
- 3 wedges of lime
- A few slices of chilli (optional)

A hearty chilli, perfectly combining the flavours of the spices with the herby lime quinoa. Refreshingly simple, colourful and appealing, this impressive dish is the ultimate comfort food to share.

1. Bring a pot of water to the boil and cook the sweet potatoes for 10 minutes until soft. Drain and set aside.

2. To make the chilli, place a pan over a medium-low heat, add the rapeseed oil, and gently cook the onion, garlic, and spices until soft. Add the canned tomatoes to the pan and simmer for 10 minutes.

3. While the chilli is cooking, prepare the quinoa, following the packet instructions. Once the quinoa is ready, season with the lime juice and zest and add half the chopped coriander.

4. Now add the cooked sweet potato, drained beans, sweetcorn, and the rest of the chopped coriander to the chilli and continue cooking over a medium-low heat until all the ingredients are heated thoroughly.

5. Divide the quinoa into three large bowls and add the bean chilli. Garnish with avocado, pumpkin seeds, lime wedge, fresh coriander, and slices of chilli.

SPICY FISH WRAP WITH COLESLAW

SERVES TWO

cod fillet loins, 2 x the size and thickness of your palm, cut into cubes
½ tsp ground allspice
½ tsp dried mixed herbs
pinch of cayenne pepper
pinch of cinnamon
pinch of ground white pepper
1 tsp extra virgin olive oil
2 wholemeal or sweet potato tortilla wraps

FOR THE GUACAMOLE

1 avocado
½ lime
½ garlic clove, crushed (optional)
bunch of fresh, chopped coriander (cilantro)
sprinkle of chilli flakes

FOR THE CRUNCHY COLESLAW

small handful of red cabbage, shredded
1 tsp fresh, chopped coriander (cilantro)
½ red onion, finely chopped
½ fresh red chilli, deseeded and finely chopped
juice of ¼ orange
2 tsp full-fat Greek yogurt OR Greek-style soya-based vegan yogurt

This dish is a combination of colours and textures. The wrap overflows with crunchy coleslaw and the burst of citrus you get from the orange works beautifully with the spicy cod and fresh avocado in the guacamole. This is not your usual wrap so give it a try!

1. If you wish to cook the fish in the oven, preheat it to 180°C (160°C fan/350°F/Gas 4).

2. Make the guacamole by crushing the avocado with a fork and squeezing the lime juice over the top. Add the garlic, coriander, and chilli flakes, mixing well. Put the guacamole in the fridge for later.

3. Put all the coleslaw ingredients in a bowl and mix thoroughly. Place in the fridge.

4. Combine the fish, allspice, mixed herbs, cayenne pepper, cinnamon, white pepper, and olive oil in a bowl. Make sure the fish is covered with all the herbs and spices but be careful not to flake the fish, try to keep it whole.

5. Gently fry the fish for approximately 10 minutes in a non-stick frying pan on a medium heat, turning halfway. Alternatively, to cook the fish in the oven, transfer it to an ovenproof dish and place in the oven for 10 minutes or until cooked through.

6. When the fish is ready, divide it into two and use it to fill the wraps with the guacamole and coleslaw.

PEKING FLATBREAD WITH SWEET CHILLI SAUCE

SERVES ONE

- chicken breast, the size and thickness of your palm, cut into cubes
- ½ tsp Chinese five spice
- 1 tsp extra virgin olive oil
- 1–2 closed cup (button) mushrooms, thinly sliced
- ½ spring (green) onion, sliced thinly
- ½ garlic clove, crushed
- ½ fresh red chilli, finely sliced
- 1 wholemeal flatbread
- few lettuce leaves
- 1 slice of beef tomato, cut in half

FOR THE SWEET CHILLI SAUCE

- 1 beef tomato
- ¼ fresh mango, peeled and stone removed
- ½ small red onion
- ½ tsp dried oregano
- small handful of fresh coriander (cilantro)
- juice of 1 lime
- juice of ½ lemon
- 1 small fresh red chilli (deseeded if you don't want it too hot)
- 1 garlic clove, crushed
- 1 tsp tomato paste

Chinese five spice is an extraordinary medley of aromatic spices that brings a punchy flavour to chicken or vegan chicken. Made from fennel seeds, cinnamon, cloves, star anise, and Szechwan peppercorns, it turns a plain stuffed flatbread into a sweet, savoury and slightly spicy, Peking-delight!

1. Blitz all the chilli sauce ingredients in a blender and put to one side.
2. Coat the chicken breast in the Chinese five spice. Heat the olive oil in a non-stick frying pan on a medium heat, then add the chicken and cook for 8–10 minutes. Now add the mushrooms, spring onion, garlic, and chilli.
3. When it's all softened and the chicken is cooked through, remove the pan from the heat. Fill the flatbread with the lettuce, tomato, and the spicy chicken mixture and top with a tablespoon of the sweet chilli sauce (or to taste).

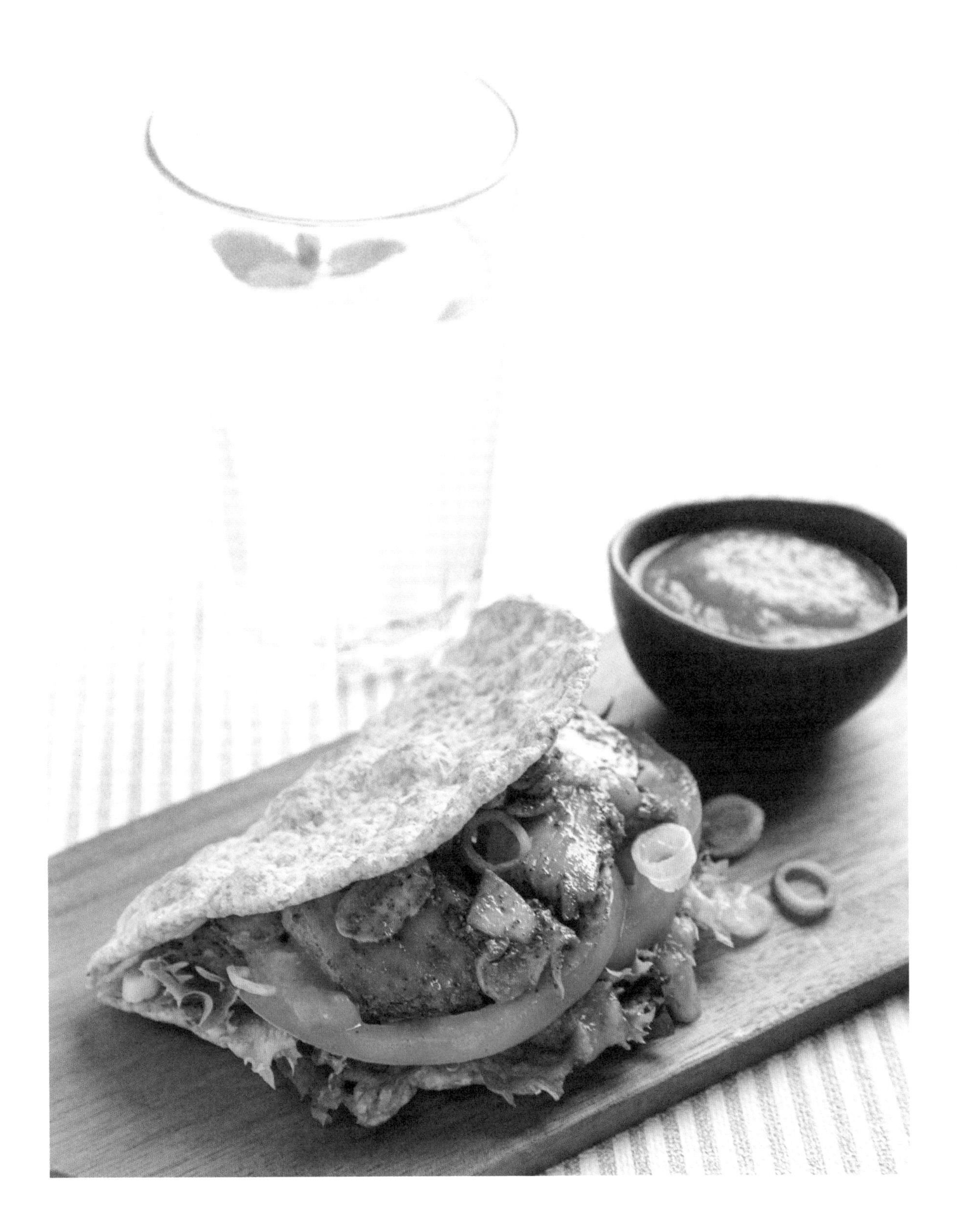

LENTIL AND SWEET POTATO CAKES WITH A SPICY MINT SAUCE

SERVES ONE

- handful of sweet potato, peeled and cut into cubes
- 1 tsp ground fennel seeds
- 400g (14oz) can of lentils, drained and rinsed
- 1 tsp extra virgin olive oil

FOR THE SPICY MINT SAUCE

- handful of fresh, chopped coriander (cilantro)
- handful of fresh, chopped mint
- juice and zest of ½ lemon
- ½ tsp cumin seeds
- 1 fresh green chilli, deseeded and chopped
- 1 garlic clove, crushed
- 2 spring (green) onions, chopped
- 3 tbsp full-fat Greek yogurt OR Greek-style soya-based vegan yogurt

TO SERVE

- small handful of mixed salad

These cakes are so delicious and perfect for lunch on the go! The addition of the warm, sweet-flavoured fennel seeds adds so much depth to the cakes, act as a powerful antioxidant and are great to keeping your heart healthy. For the freshest flavour, you can grind the fennel seeds either in a pestle and mortar or in a bowl using the end of a rolling pin.

1. Preheat the oven to 180°C (160°C fan/350°F/Gas 4).
2. Add the sweet potato to a pan of boiling water and boil for around 10 minutes until soft, then drain and set aside.
3. Add the ground fennel seeds to the cooked potato with the lentils and mash everything together.
4. Divide the mixture in half and shape into two patties.
5. Use half of the oil to grease your baking tray, then coat the cakes with the remaining oil and cook for 30–40 minutes, turning halfway through.
6. Meanwhile, make the spicy mint sauce by putting all the ingredients into a blender and blitzing.
7. To serve, transfer the cakes to a plate, drizzle with the spicy mint sauce, and serve with a small mixed salad.

GOOD TO KNOW

Put the spicy mint sauce in an airtight container and it will last in the fridge for a few days or, alternatively, you can freeze it in a couple of separate freezer bags and it will last a month.

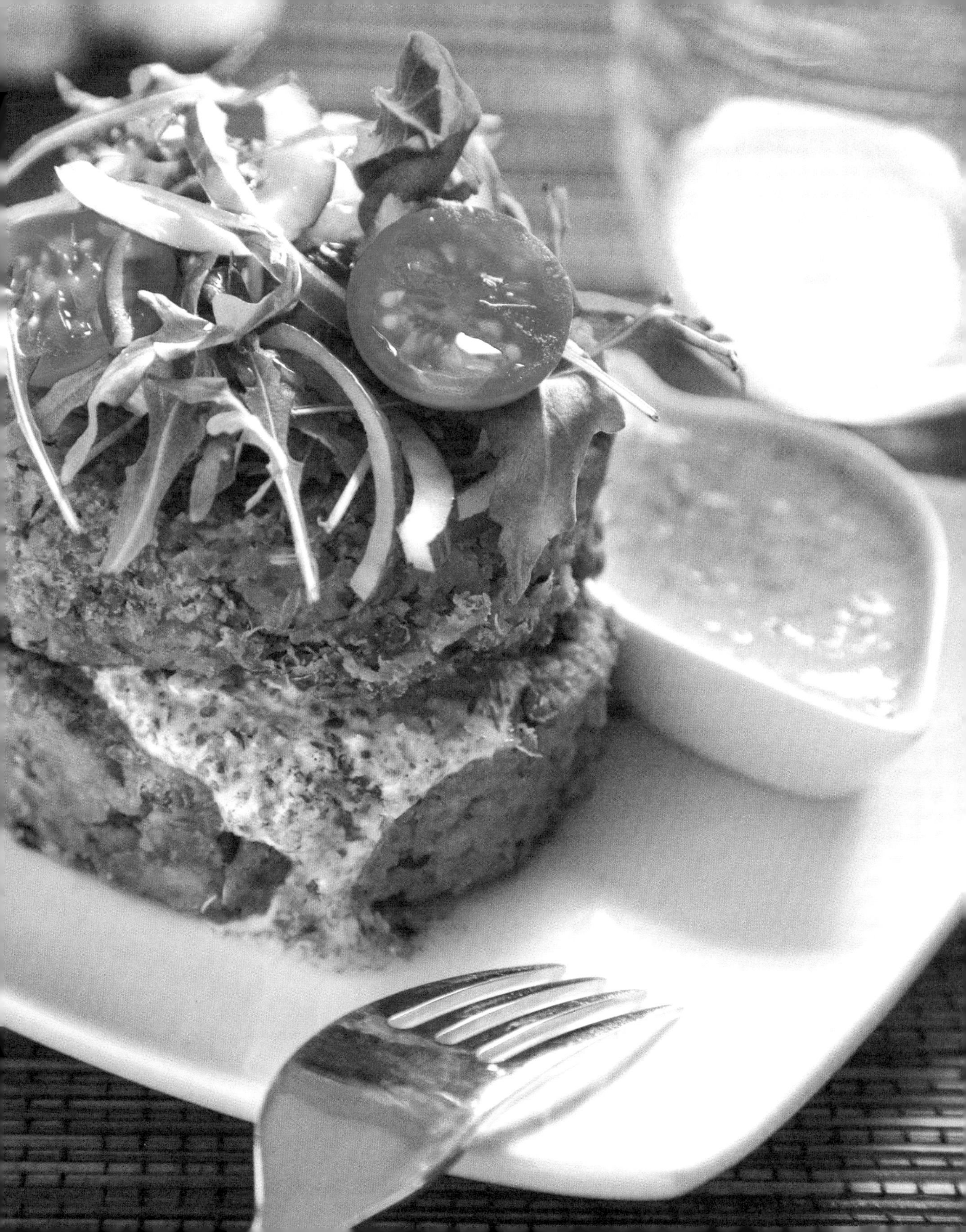

TOM YUM FRAGRANT CHICKEN SOUP

SERVES TWO

- 2 tsp coconut oil
- ½ white onion chopped
- ½ fennel bulb
- ½ celery stalk, chopped
- 1 small courgette (zucchini), chopped
- small handful of green beans, chopped
- 1 tsp fennel seeds
- 1 bay leaf
- 1 lemongrass stalk, bashed to release its flavour
- 1 fresh red chilli (deseeded if you do not like it too hot)
- 1 tsp curry leaves
- 1 star anise
- 1 garlic clove, crushed
- 2 chicken breasts, the size and thickness of your palm, cut into cubes
- juice and zest of 1 lemon
- juice and zest of 1 lime
- handful of fresh, chopped coriander (cilantro)

Fresh and fragrant, Thai soups range from rich, creamy coconut to hot clear broths. Besides being the most famous of all Thai soups, *tom yum* offers many health benefits due to its potent combination of herbs and spices. Truly delicious, this easy soup has the desired punch in both flavour and nutritional value.

1. In a medium to large non-stick pan, heat the coconut oil and stir-fry all the ingredients apart from the chicken, coriander, lemon, and lime for around 8 minutes.
2. Add the chicken, lemon, and lime zest to the pan and stir-fry until the chicken is sealed.
3. Cover the ingredients of the pan with boiling water and simmer for 20–30 minutes.
4. When you have 5 minutes left, add the lemon and lime juice and stir well.
5. Serve in bowls and garnish with some fresh coriander.

WHITE BEAN AND TOFU RATATOUILLE

SERVES TWO

- 400g (14oz) can of chopped tomatoes
- ½ red onion, roughly chopped
- 2 garlic cloves, chopped
- 1 tbsp dried oregano
- 1 handful button (closed cup) mushrooms, sliced
- 1 tbsp smoked paprika
- 1 tsp ground white pepper
- 400g (14oz) can of butter (lima) beans, drained and rinsed
- large handful of sliced aubergine (eggplant) and courgette (zucchini)
- 10 fresh basil leaves
- silken tofu, 1½ x the size and thickness of your palm
- 1 tsp extra virgin olive oil
- 6 pitted black olives, sliced
- freshly ground black pepper

Ratatouille originates from the Provence region in France and was created as a side dish to make the most of garden vegetables. My healthy and balanced recipe, with the addition of the slightly sweet and nutty silken tofu and sumptuous white beans, elevates it from the side-lines to centre stage.

1. Preheat the oven to 180°C (160°C fan/350°F/Gas 4).
2. Add the chopped tomatoes, onion, garlic, oregano, mushrooms, paprika, white pepper, and 200ml (scant 1 cup) of water to a medium pan over a medium heat. Bring to the boil, then reduce the heat and simmer for 10 minutes. Add the beans, stir well, and turn off the heat.
3. Cover the base of a small ovenproof dish with half the aubergine and courgette slices. Next, spoon over half the tomato and bean mixture before evenly spreading the basil leaves on top.
4. Spoon over a second layer of aubergine and courgette followed by the remaining tomato and bean mixture.
5. Add the silken tofu, olive oil, and sliced black olives to a mixing bowl and roughly mix with a fork, then generously spoon the mixture over the ratatouille and season with a good grinding of pepper.
6. Place the dish in the preheated oven and bake for 20 minutes.

CRAB CAKES WITH COLESLAW

SERVES ONE

- handful of sweet potato, peeled and cut into cubes
- canned or fresh white crab meat, the size and thickness of your palm (if canned then squeeze out excess water)
- ½ spring (green) onion, finely chopped
- ½ mild fresh red chilli, deseeded and finely chopped
- zest of 1 lime (reserve a wedge for serving)
- 1 tsp extra virgin olive oil
- 1 heaped tsp fresh, chopped coriander (cilantro)

FOR THE CRUNCHY COLESLAW

- small handful of red cabbage, shredded
- 1 tsp fresh, chopped coriander (cilantro)
- ½ red onion, finely chopped
- ½ fresh red chilli, deseeded and finely chopped
- juice of ¼ orange
- 2 tsp full-fat Greek yogurt OR Greek-style soya-based vegan yogurt

TO SERVE

- a few green leaves
- 1 tbsp full-fat Greek yogurt OR Greek-style soya-based vegan yogurt
- a couple of fresh mint leaves, finely chopped

Rich crab meat is perfectly complemented here by the tangy cool and aromatic minty yogurt. This is a quick and delicious midweek meal rich in omega-3 fatty acids and is perfect for health-conscious foodies.

1. Preheat the oven to 180°C (160°C fan/350°F/Gas 4) and line a baking tray with foil.
2. Make the minty yogurt sauce to serve. Place the yogurt in a small bowl and combine with the mint leaves. Leave to one side.
3. Bring a pan of water to the boil and cook the sweet potato for approximately 10 minutes, or until soft. Then drain and mash the potato and leave to cool.
4. Combine the crab meat, spring onion, chilli, lime zest, olive oil, and fresh coriander in a bowl.
5. Add the sweet potato mash to the crab mixture, combine thoroughly, and shape into 3 small patties.
6. Transfer the crab cakes to the baking tray and cook in the oven for approximately 20 minutes until cooked through. Meanwhile, prepare your coleslaw by adding the ingredients to a bowl and mixing thoroughly, then set to one side.
7. Serve your crab cakes on a plate with some leaves, coleslaw, and a tablespoon of the minty yogurt.

GOOD TO KNOW

Put the minty yogurt in an airtight container and it will last in the fridge for a few days or, alternatively, you can freeze it in a couple of separate freezer bags and it will last a month.

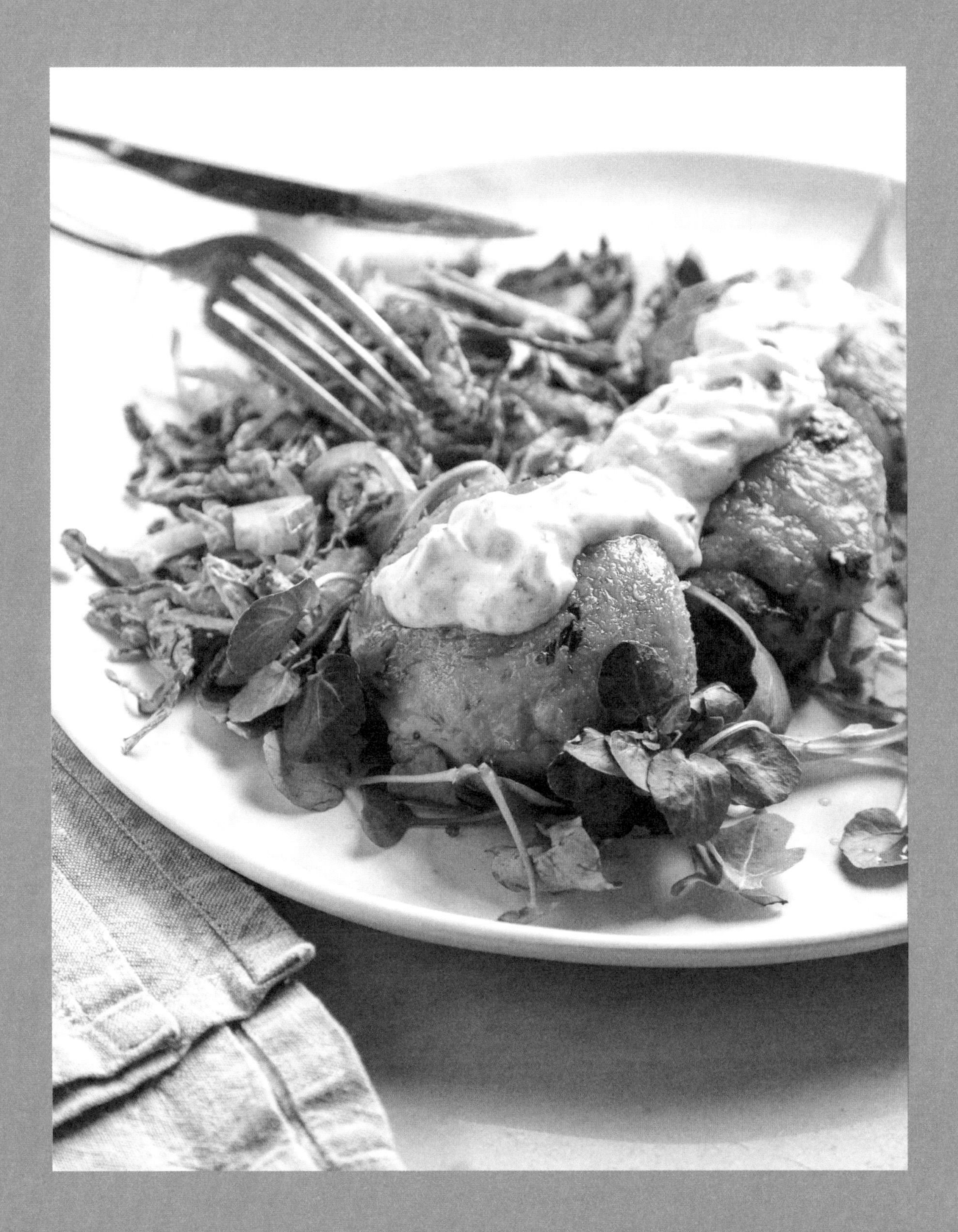

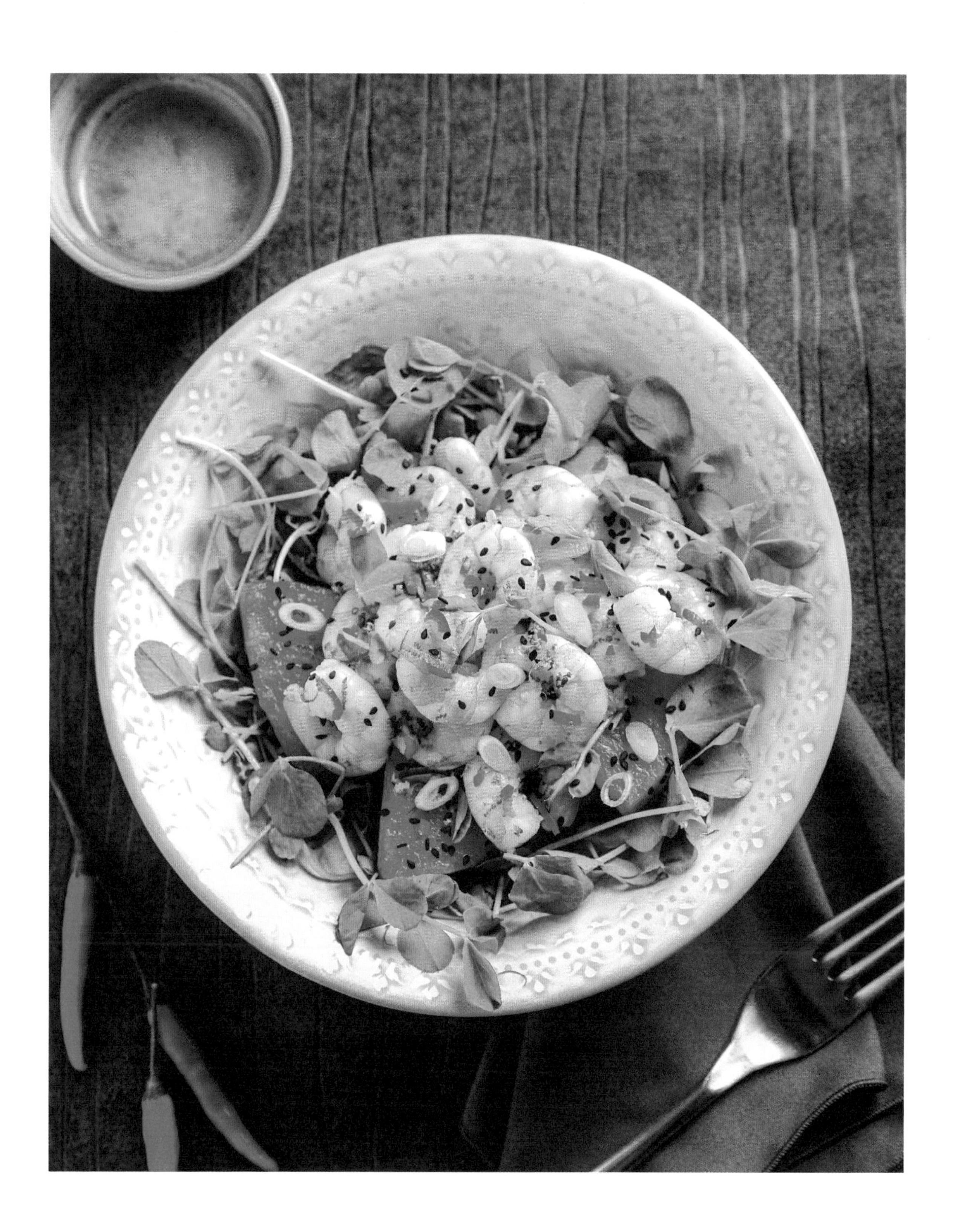

CHILLI AND LIME KING PRAWN WITH WATERMELON SALAD

SERVES ONE

- king prawns, cooked and peeled, the size and thickness of your palm
- zest of ½ lime
- handful of green leafy salad leaves
- wedge of watermelon, chopped
- 1 spring (green) onion, finely sliced
- sprinkle of black sesame seeds (optional)

FOR THE DRESSING

- 1 garlic clove, crushed
- juice of ½ lime
- ½ fresh red chilli, finely chopped
- 1 tsp extra virgin olive oil

Nothing says summer as much as this recipe. Watermelon is the quintessential fruit of summer, and its sweet flavour is well matched with the lime and chilli in this recipe.

1. Start by making the dressing. Mix the crushed garlic, lime juice, chilli, and olive oil in a small dish and leave to one side ready for serving.
2. Toss the prawns in the lime zest to coat.
3. Now start layering the salad. Line a medium serving bowl with the salad leaves. Add the chopped watermelon and top with the zesty lime prawns. Sprinkle with the spring onion and black sesame seeds.
4. Drizzle over the dressing and serve.

MARINATED TOFU AND APPLE SALAD

SERVES ONE

- extra firm tofu, 1½ x the size and thickness of your palm, cut into cubes
- large handful of baby spinach leaves
- ¼ avocado, sliced
- ¼ green apple, sliced
- 1 tbsp raisins

FOR THE DRESSING

- ½ tsp extra virgin olive oil
- 1 thumb-size piece of fresh ginger root, grated
- juice of ½ lemon
- small handful of fresh, chopped flat-leaf parsley

FOR THE MARINADE

- 1 tsp sumac
- zest of 1 lemon
- small handful of fresh, chopped coriander (cilantro)
- 1 tbsp full-fat Greek yogurt OR Greek-style soya-based vegan yogurt

This is a salad made up of perfect partners. Avocado and spinach, lemon and ginger. I've also added sumac to my marinade, although a less common spice, it brings a pleasant tangy vibe with a hint of citrus fruitiness to my tofu!

1. Preheat the oven to 180°C (160°C fan/350°F/Gas 4).
2. Add all the dressing ingredients to a small bowl, whisk, and set aside.
3. In a mixing bowl, add all the marinade ingredients and stir thoroughly. Add the tofu and combine until the tofu pieces are completely coated.
4. Place the tofu cubes on a non-stick baking tray and bake for 10 minutes or until they start to bubble or turn a nice brown colour.
5. In a bowl, add the spinach leaves and avocado, top with the baked tofu, apple slices, sprinkle with raisins and drizzle the zesty dressing all over.

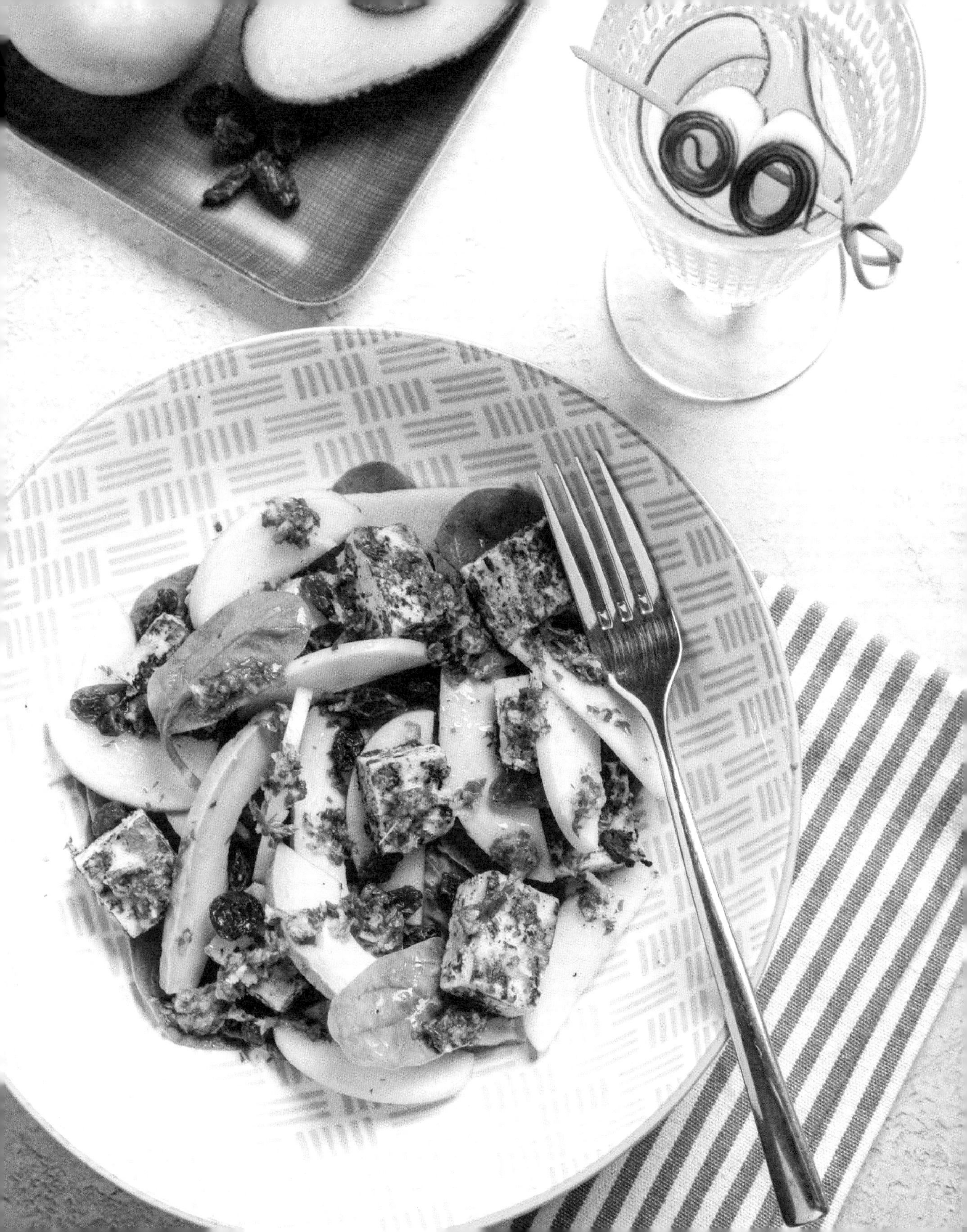

HERBY SARDINES WITH TABBOULEH

SERVES ONE

- 1 tsp fresh, finely chopped rosemary
- 1 tsp finely fresh, chopped flat-leaf parsley
- 1 garlic clove, crushed
- 3 pitted black or green olives, finely chopped
- juice and zest of 1 lemon
- pinch of ground white pepper
- ½ tsp extra virgin olive oil
- 4 fresh sardines, gutted and cleaned

FOR THE TABBOULEH

- 2 tbsp bulgur wheat dry weight (6 tbsp cooked weight)
- 2 tbsp chopped, flat-leaf parsley
- 2 tomatoes, finely chopped
- 1 tbsp fresh, chopped mint
- 3 spring onions, finely chopped
- juice of ½ lemon
- 1 tsp extra virgin olive oil
- ¼ tsp ground allspice
- ¼ tsp sumac
- freshly ground black pepper

I love going to the fishmonger and selecting my fresh sardines. If they are not already prepared, remember to ask your fishmonger to gut and clean them for you. Definitely give this recipe a try as it's one of my all-time favourites. I like to remove the fish bones, but you can cook the fish whole and eat the soft bones, if you prefer.

1. Mix the rosemary, parsley, garlic, olives, lemon juice and zest, white pepper, and olive oil together in a bowl to create a herby mixture.

2. To make the tabbouleh, cook the bulgur wheat following the packet instructions, drain, and leave to cool. Mix the bulgur wheat in a bowl with all the other ingredients and season with the black pepper.

3. If you want to remove the bones from the sardines, turn the fish skin-side up and press down firmly along the backbone. Turn the fish back over and pull out the backbone, then cut it off with a pair of scissors. If any small bones remain you can remove them with tweezers. Next, rub the herby zesty mixture generously over both sides, making sure each sardine is coated well.

4. Place the sardines on a sheet of foil under a medium grill (broiler) for 4 minutes on each side.

5. Once the fish are cooked, serve with the tabbouleh.

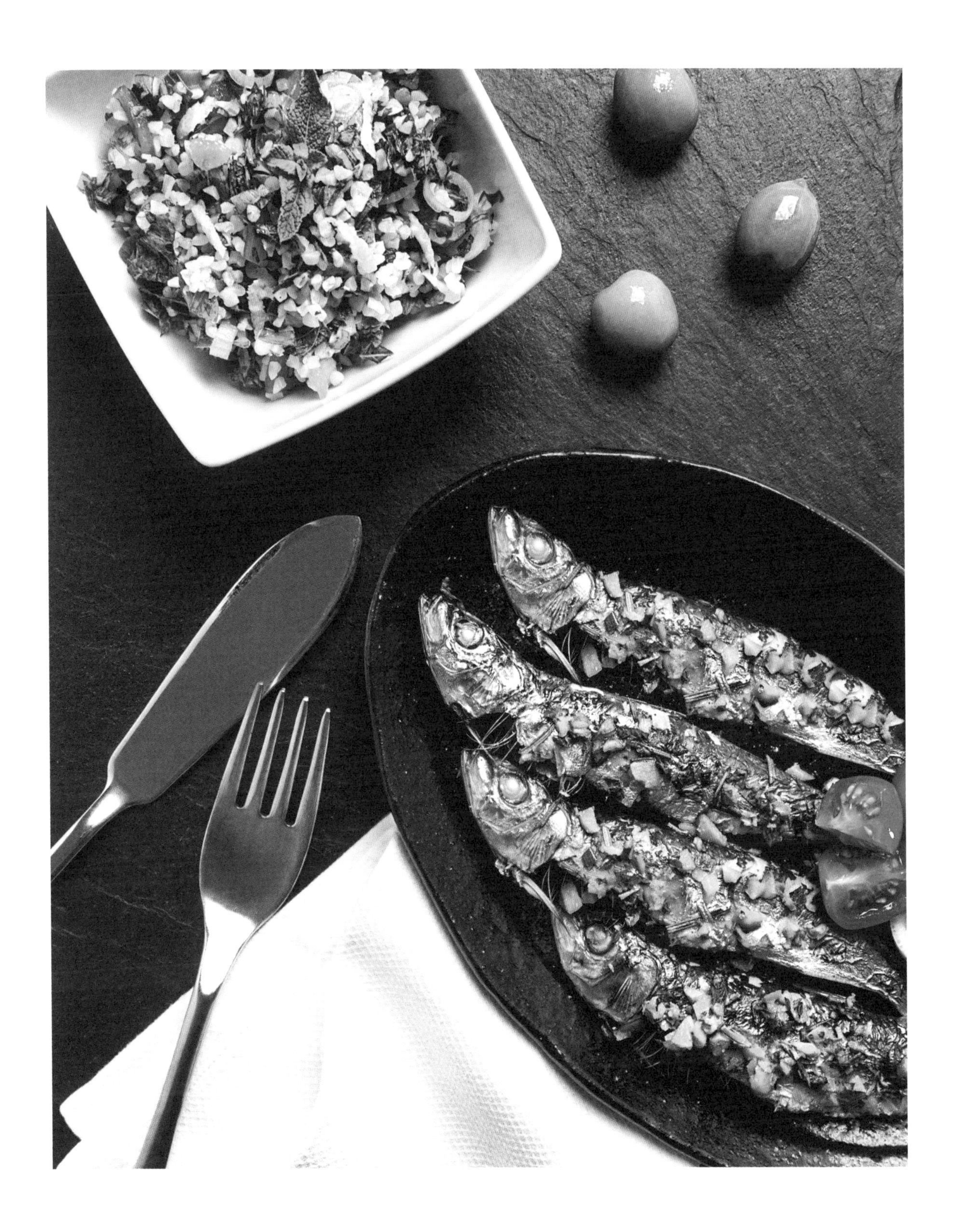

TOFU KEBABS WITH CHIMICHURRI

SERVES TWO

- firm tofu, 3 x the size and thickness of your palm, cut into cubes
- ½ courgette (zucchini), sliced
- 8 cherry tomatoes
- ½ yellow pepper, deseeded and chopped into large pieces
- 1 small red onion, chopped into large chunks
- mixed salad leaves

FOR THE CHIMICHURRI

- small handful of fresh, roughly chopped flat-leaf parsley
- small handful of fresh, roughly chopped coriander (cilantro)
- 1 tsp dried oregano
- 2 garlic cloves, roughly chopped
- 1 tsp smoked paprika
- ½ red chilli, deseeded and roughly chopped (optional)
- juice and zest of 1 lime

FOR THE MARINADE

- 2 tsp extra virgin olive oil
- juice and zest of 1 orange
- ½ tsp ground white pepper
- 1 tsp tomato paste
- 1 tsp paprika
- 1 tsp garlic powder
- 1 tsp onion powder
- 1 tsp ground cumin
- 1 tsp dried oregano

Chimichurri, a vibrant and flavourful sauce hailing from Latin America, is the ideal partner to my spiced tofu kebabs. This bright green, smoky sauce enhances the kebabs perfectly so let the flavours mingle as you marinate this dish to perfection!

1. To make the chimichurri, put all ingredients in a blender along with 50ml (3⅓ tablespoons) of water and blitz. Transfer to a bowl and store in the fridge until later.
2. Meanwhile, preheat the grill (broiler) to medium. If using wooden skewers (rather than metal ones), soak them in some water in the sink or a bowl so they do not burn when you pop them under the grill.
3. Add all marinade ingredients to a mixing bowl and whisk, then toss the tofu in the marinade until fully coated. Leave to soak for 10 minutes so the tofu can take on the flavour of the marinade.
4. Build the skewers, alternating vegetables and tofu. Place them under the grill, turning frequently until they start to bubble or are turning a nice brown colour.
5. Serve the skewers on a plate with the mixed salad leaves and a good drizzle of the chimichurri dressing.

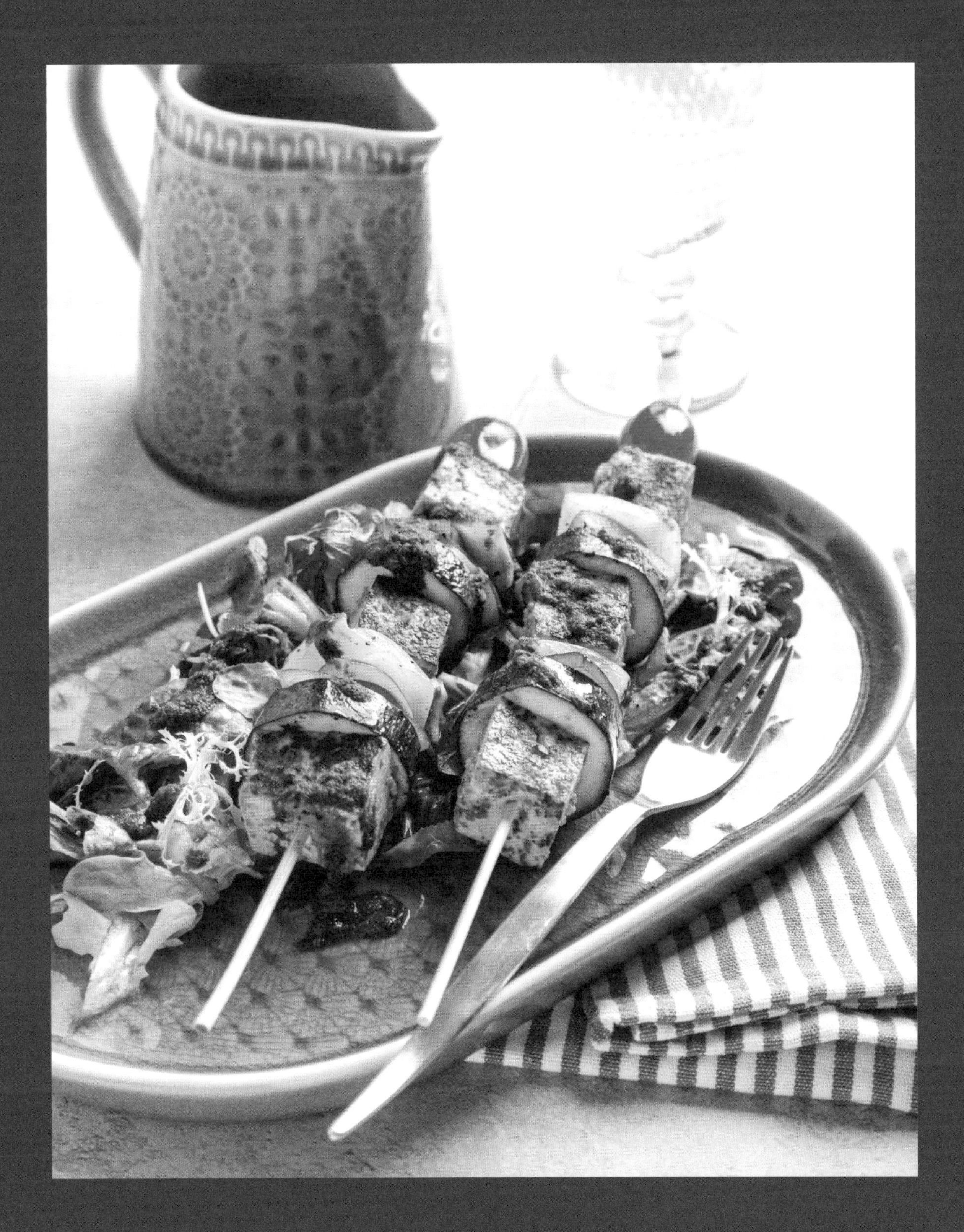

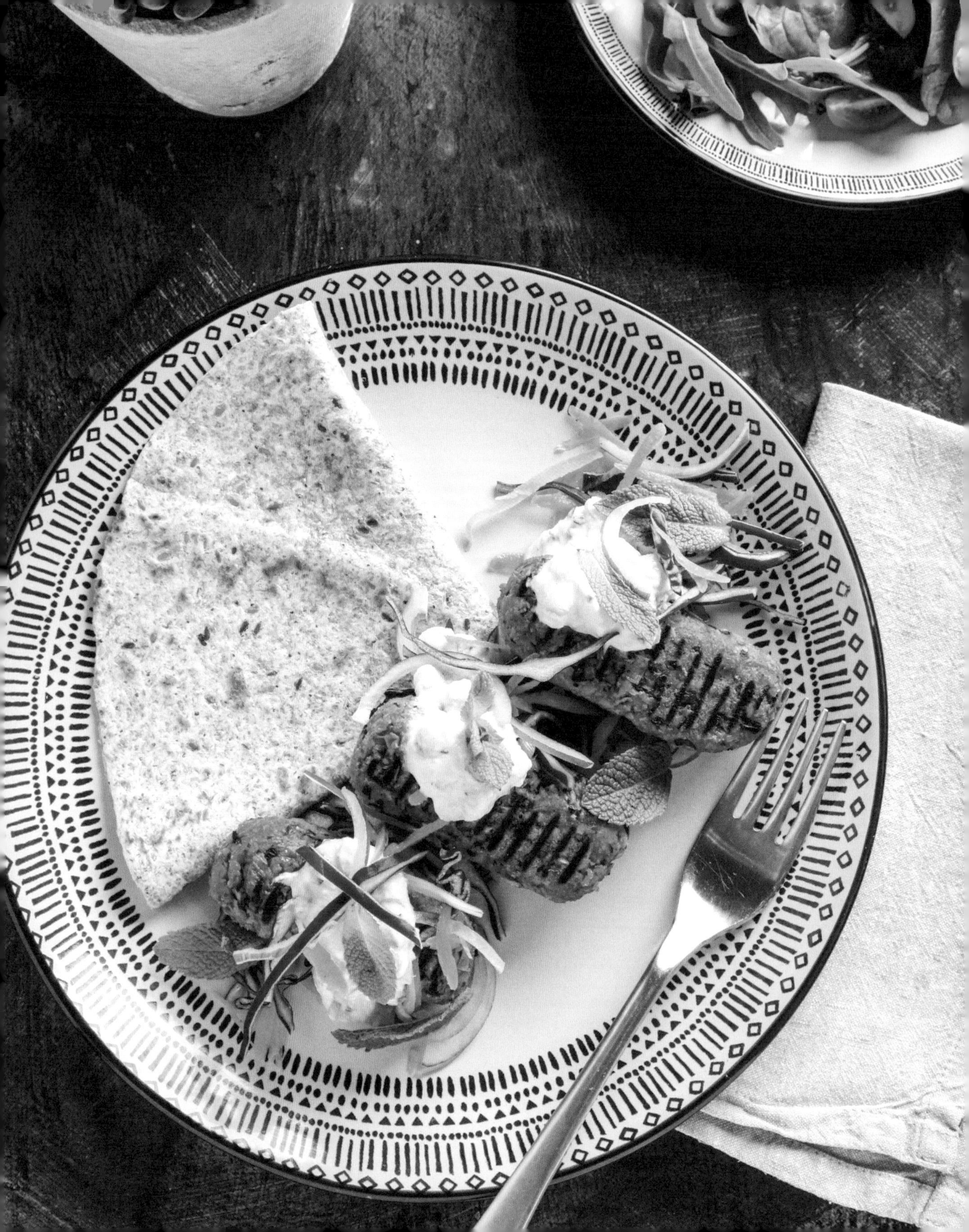

PLANT-BASED KOFTE WRAP

SERVES TWO

- 2 tsp extra virgin olive oil
- ½ white onion, diced
- 1 garlic clove, finely chopped
- 1 tsp ground cumin
- 1 tsp ground coriander
- 1 tsp cinnamon
- 1 tsp smoked paprika
- 1 tsp ground ginger
- plant-based mince (crumbles), 3 x the size and thickness of your palm
- pinch of black pepper
- handful of fresh, chopped mint and coriander (cilantro), plus a few extra mint leaves to garnish
- 2 wholemeal wraps
- green leafy salad (optional)

FOR THE SLAW

- small handful of sliced red cabbage, grated carrot, and sliced red onion
- freshly ground black pepper
- juice and zest of 1 lime

FOR THE YOGURT DRESSING

- 2 tbsp full-fat Greek yogurt OR Greek-style soya-based vegan yogurt
- 3 fresh, finely chopped mint leaves
- pinch of chilli flakes
- juice of ½ lemon
- 1 spring (green) onion, finely sliced

This mouth-watering dish is rich in vitamins, minerals and antioxidants. Deliciously warm from the spices and cool from the 'slaw and yogurt dressing, it offers a wholesome dose of goodness in every bite. A real Turkish delight!

1. Preheat the oven to 180°C (160°C fan/350°F/Gas 4).
2. In a non-stick pan, over a low to medium heat, add the olive oil, onion, garlic, and spices and cook gently until softened, then transfer to a mixing bowl.
3. Add the plant-based mince to the bowl with the onion, garlic, and herbs, and season with black pepper. Then, using your hands, shape the mixture into six sausage-shaped koftas.
4. Heat a griddle pan over a medium heat and add the koftas. Cook them for 2 minutes on each side, then transfer to a baking tray and cook in the oven for a further 10 minutes.
5. While the koftas are cooking, add the slaw ingredients to a clean mixing bowl and combine.
6. In a separate small bowl, add the yogurt dressing ingredients and mix well to combine.
7. In a frying pan, dry-fry the wraps for 10–15 seconds on both sides.
8. Place each wrap on a plate, add the koftas and slaw, then garnish with 1 tablespoon of the yogurt dressing and some of the remaining fresh mint. If you like, serve with a small handful of salad.

QUORN SALAD WITH GRIDDLED NECTARINES AND MINT

SERVES TWO

- 1 tsp extra virgin olive oil
- juice and zest of 1 lime
- 2 tbsp fresh, finely chopped mint, plus a few leaves to garnish
- 1 garlic clove, crushed
- Quorn pieces, 3 x the size and thickness of your palm
- handful of fine green beans, halved
- 2 nectarines, each cut into 8 wedges
- 1 small red onion, sliced into rings
- 1 Little Gem lettuce, shredded
- 1 small avocado, sliced
- handful of rocket (arugula)

The unexpected sweet caramelization of the griddled nectarines, paired so effortlessly with fresh mint, makes this unassuming warm salad a summer triumph! The addition of creamy avocado and peppery rocket moves it right up the line to a super salad sensation.

1. Mix the olive oil, lime juice and zest, and chopped mint in a bowl and add the garlic. Divide the mixture into two bowls, and set one aside.
2. Add the Quorn pieces to one of the bowls containing the zesty mixture, stirring them through until they are coated.
3. Place a non-stick frying pan over a low heat and add the Quorn pieces, cooking for about 5 minutes until they are warmed through.
4. Bring a small pan of water to the boil and add the green beans. Cook them for 3–4 minutes until tender.
5. At the same time, griddle the nectarines for a few minutes in a griddle pan over a high heat, turning once, until slightly charred.
6. Drain the beans and toss them with the red onion in the remaining portion of the lime, mint and garlic mixture.
7. To serve, layer the salad into two bowls, starting with the lettuce and some of the rocket, then the beans and onions, followed by the Quorn pieces. Add the griddled nectarine slices, avocado, rocket, and garnish with the remaining mint leaves.

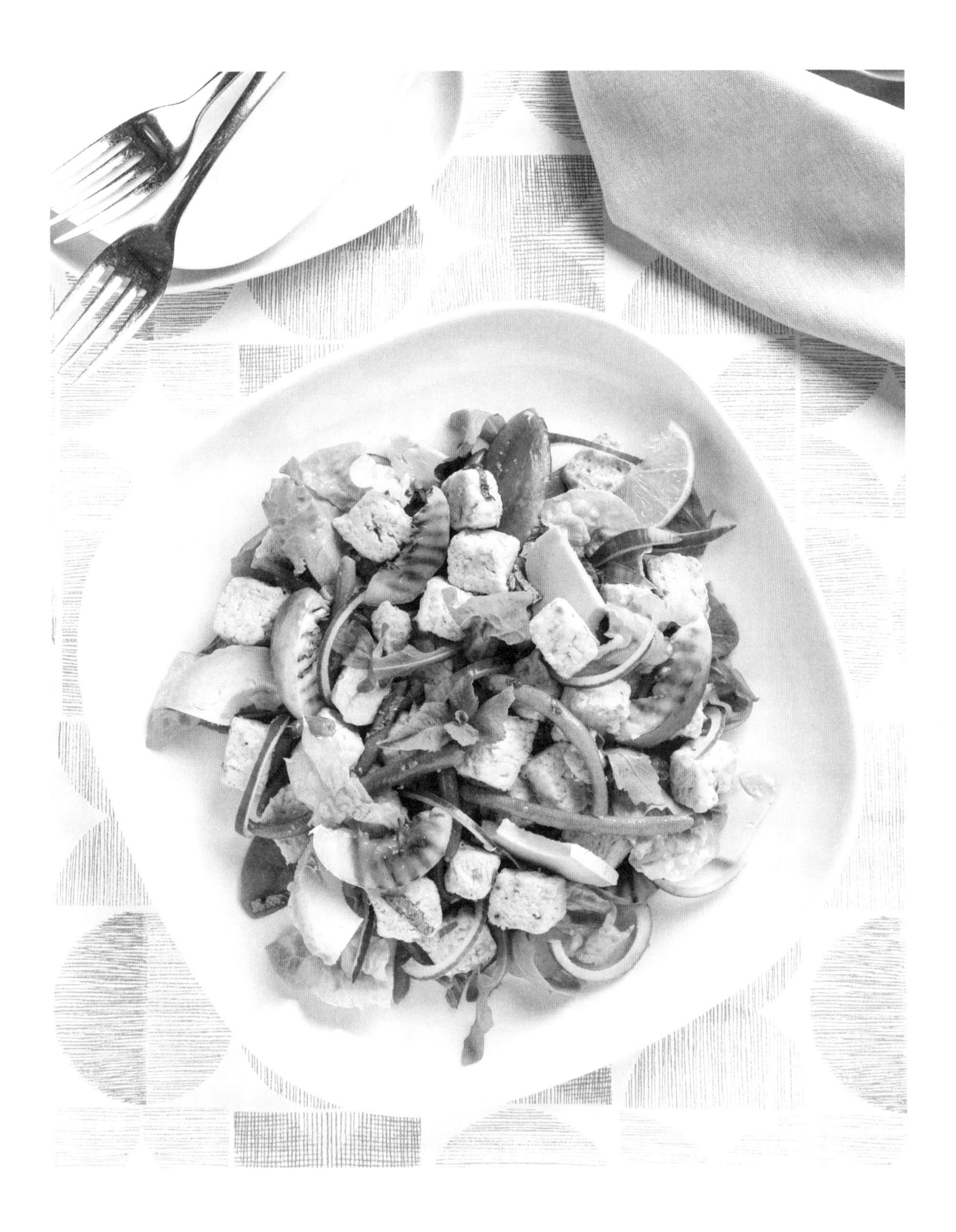

CHERMOULA CHICKEN WITH PAPAYA

SERVES ONE

- 1 chicken breast, the size and thickness of your palm, cut into cubes
- 1 tsp extra virgin olive oil
- 3–4 Little Gem lettuce leaves, or similar
- ¼ cucumber, finely chopped
- ½ small red onion, finely sliced
- ¼ papaya, finely chopped
- pinch of chilli flakes

FOR THE MARINADE

- juice and zest of ½ lemon
- ½ tsp ground cumin
- ½ tsp ground coriander
- 1 heaped tsp fresh, chopped coriander (cilantro), save a little for a garnish
- 1 heaped tsp fresh, chopped flat-leaf parsley
- ½ tsp paprika

I've taken North Africa's most popular marinade, the delicious chermoula, and paired it with the fat-burning, vitamin-rich, healing papaya. Deliciously sweet with soft flesh, papaya is known to be one of the world's healthiest fruits, so it is a perfect accompaniment to any of my healthy recipes.

1. Make the marinade by combining the lemon juice and zest, cumin, ground and fresh coriander, parsley, and paprika in a bowl.
2. Add the chicken, mix well, cover with cling film (plastic wrap) and either leave in the fridge overnight or move on to step 3.
3. Add the olive oil to a non-stick frying pan and slowly cook the chicken on a medium heat for 10–15 minutes, or until completely cooked through.
4. Place the lettuce leaves on a plate, divide the cucumber, cooked chicken, sliced red onion, and papaya between the leaves.
5. Sprinkle with a few chilli flakes, garnish with fresh coriander, and enjoy.

GOOD TO KNOW

If you can't get hold of papaya you can use mango instead. I like to prep the chicken and leave it covered in the fridge overnight to absorb the delicious flavours of the marinade. If you're short on time you can skip this step and it will be just as delicious.

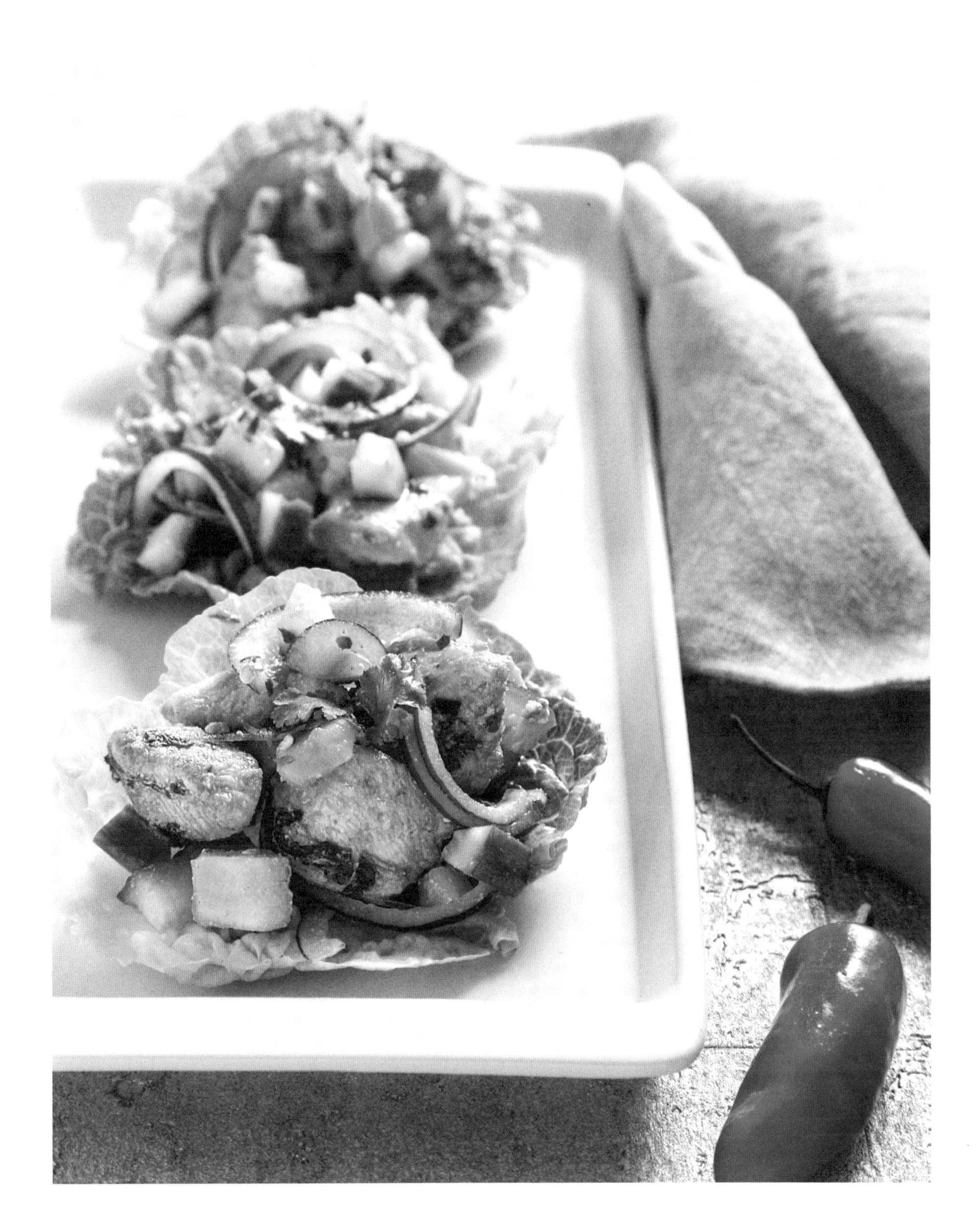

ORANGE AND GINGER TEMPEH

SERVES FOUR

- tempeh, 6 x the size and thickness of your palm, cut into finger size strips
- 1 head of pak choi (bok choy), stalk removed
- handful of baby corn
- handful of green beans
- handful of tenderstem broccoli (broccolini)
- 4 tsp sesame oil
- 2 tbsp sesame seeds
- 1 orange, peeled and segmented
- handful of fresh coriander (cilantro) leaves

FOR THE MARINADE

- juice and zest of 2 oranges
- 2 fresh red chillies, deseeded and finely chopped
- 1 heaped tsp grated fresh ginger root
- 5 garlic cloves, crushed
- handful of fresh, chopped basil

This dish is all about the tempeh. This meat alternative, made from soya beans (soybeans) absorbs flavour easily, so it's perfect for the sticky orange, chilli, ginger, and fragrant basil marinade.

1. Add the marinade ingredients to a mixing bowl and stir well, then stir in the sliced tempeh until coated.
2. Bring a pot of water to the boil. Once boiling, add all the vegetables for 1 minute, then drain.
3. Heat a non-stick frying pan, add the sesame oil and over a medium heat add the pieces of tempeh (reserve any excess marinade). Cook the tempeh on both sides for 1 minute until golden.
4. Now add all vegetables and sesame seeds to the same pan and stir-fry for 2 minutes with any excess marinade.
5. Serve in large bowls and garnish with orange segments and fresh coriander.

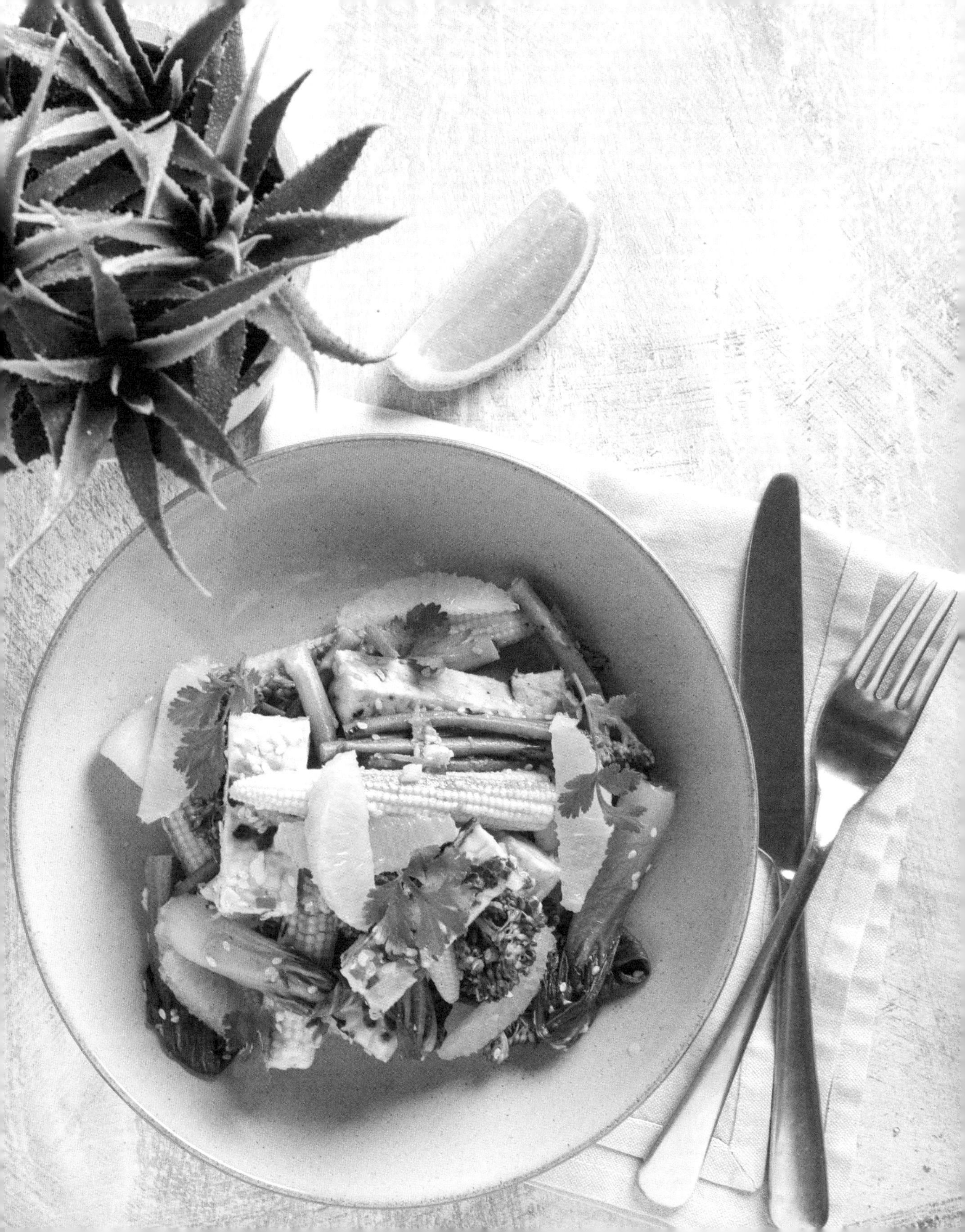

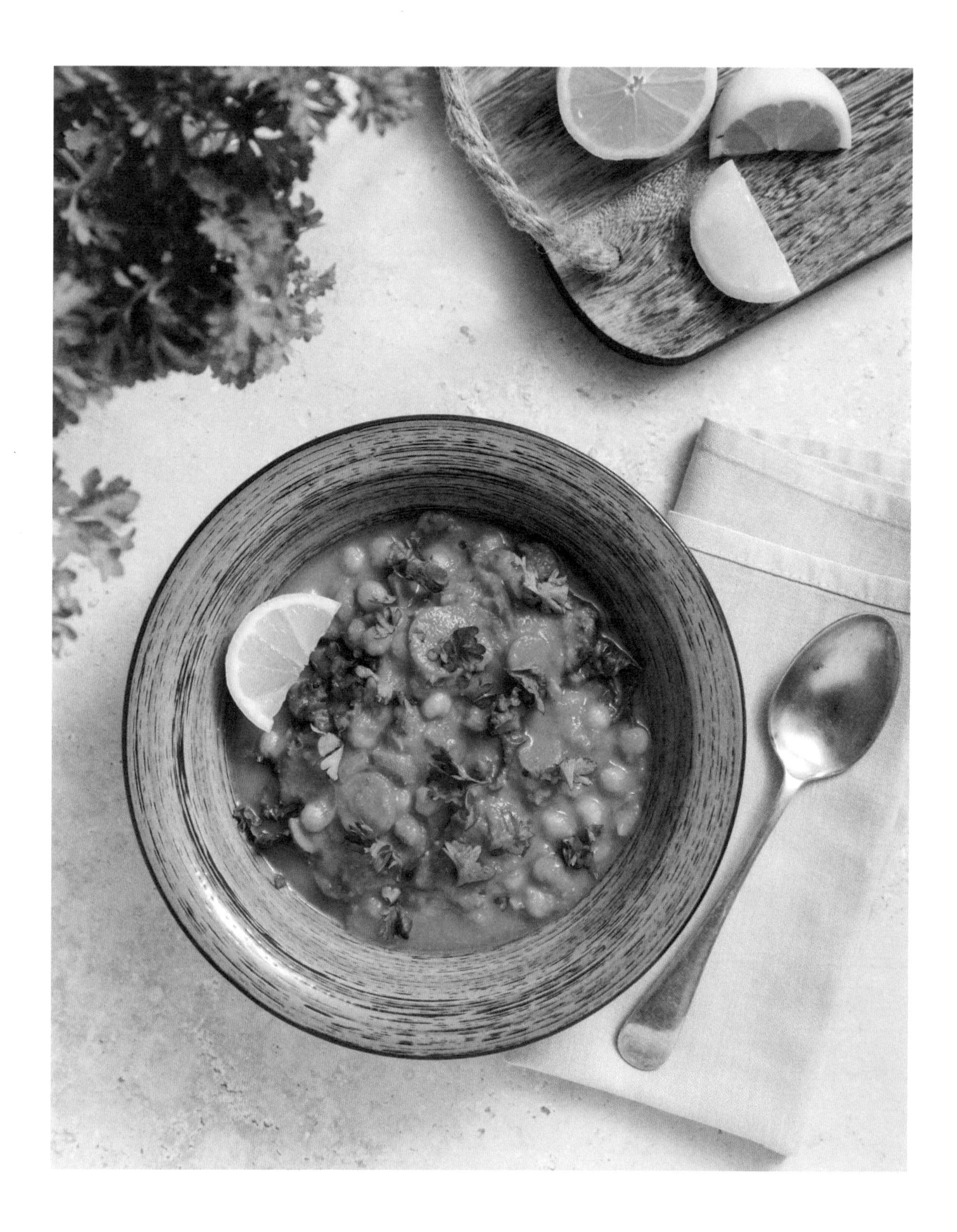

TUSCAN STEW

SERVES TWO

- 1 tsp extra virgin olive oil
- ½ combined handful of sliced carrot, celery, and red onion
- 4 garlic cloves, roughly chopped
- 1 tsp smoked paprika
- 1 tsp ground cumin
- 1 tsp dried thyme
- 1 tsp fresh, chopped rosemary
- ½ tsp ground white pepper
- 1 tsp tomato paste
- 2 x 400g (14oz) cans of chickpeas, drained and rinsed
- ½ can (200g/7oz) of chopped tomatoes
- 1 bay leaf
- handful of chopped kale (stalks removed)
- 6 pitted green or black olives, sliced

TO SERVE

- juice of ½ lemon
- a few fresh, chopped flat-leaf parsley leaves
- lemon wedge

This easy-to-make hearty bean stew is packed with the flavours of Tuscany. It is so warm and nourishing, with the added benefit of a vitamin hit courtesy of the kale and antioxidant-rich olives.

1. Heat the olive oil in a pan and gently fry the carrot, celery, onion, garlic, spices and herbs (excluding the bay leaf) over a low heat for 5 minutes. Add the white pepper and tomato paste and cook for a further minute.

2. Now add the chickpeas, 500ml (generous 2 cups) of water, the chopped tomatoes, and bay leaf. Turn up the heat and bring to the boil, then simmer for 10 minutes. Remove the pan from the heat and leave to cool for a few minutes.

3. Remove the bay leaf and transfer half the stew to a blender and blitz for 1 minute. Open the blender (with caution!) and return the blended mixture to the rest of the stew in the pan.

4. Put the pan back over a medium heat, add the kale and olives, bring to the boil before serving. Ladle the stew into two large bowls, stir in the lemon juice and garnish with some freshly chopped parsley and a wedge of lemon.

CHICKEN PESTO SALAD

SERVES ONE

- 1 chicken breast, the size and thickness of your palm, cut into cubes
- mixed leaf salad
- few ribbons of courgette (zucchini)
- few slices of red onion
- wedge of lemon

FOR THE PESTO

- ½ bunch of fresh basil
- 5 tsp extra virgin olive oil
- 6 almonds
- 2 garlic cloves, crushed
- juice of ½ lemon
- freshly ground black pepper

What is it about pesto that makes every dish leap off the plate into your mouth? You can pretty much add it to anything, but if you want to stay healthy then stick to giving your chicken and salads a gorgeous treat of this fresh garlicky basil paste.

1. Prepare the pesto by adding all the ingredients to a food processor and blitzing.
2. Place the chicken in a bowl. Marinate by rubbing 1 heaped teaspoon of pesto into the chicken with the back of a spoon. Refrigerate, covered, for half an hour or overnight if possible.
3. Preheat the oven to 180°C (160°C fan/350°F/Gas 4). Transfer the marinated chicken to a baking tray and place in the oven for approximately 20 minutes or until cooked through.
4. Remove the chicken from the oven, leave to cool slightly and serve with the salad leaves, courgette, red onion, and the wedge of lemon.

GOOD TO KNOW

Put the pesto in an airtight container and it will last in the fridge for a few days or, alternatively, you can freeze it in a couple of separate freezer bags and it will last a month.

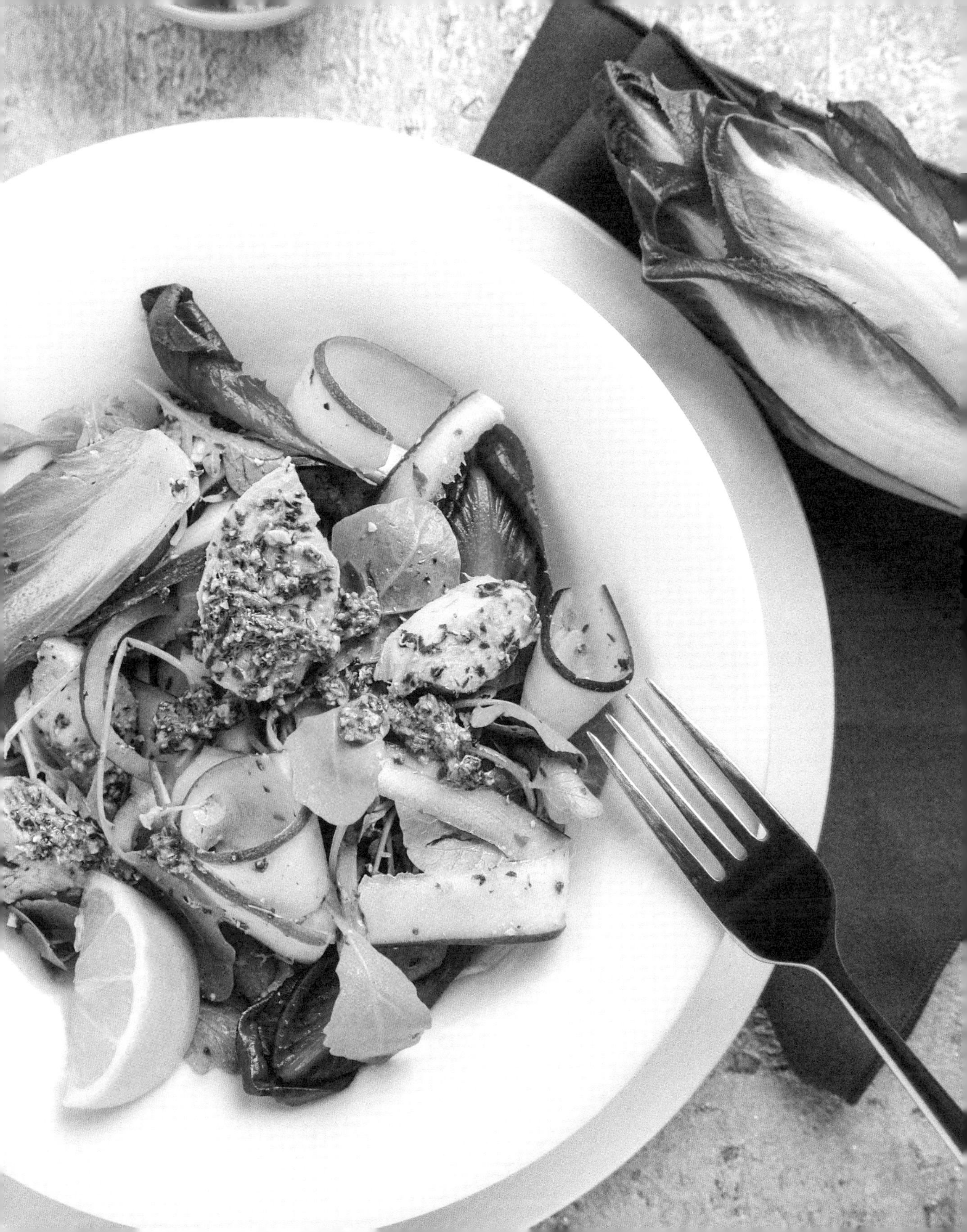

CHICKEN BREAST IN A ROASTED RED PEPPER SAUCE

SERVES ONE

- 1 handful size of sweet potato
- 1 chicken breast, the size and thickness of your palm
- ½ tsp extra virgin olive oil
- freshly ground black pepper
- pinch of dried mixed herbs
- 1 tbsp full-fat cottage cheese OR full-fat Greek yogurt OR Greek-style soya-based vegan yogurt

FOR THE SAUCE

- ½ red pepper, deseeded and roughly chopped
- ½ red onion, roughly chopped
- 1 garlic clove, whole
- 3 pitted black or green olives
- 10 fresh basil leaves
- 1 tsp tomato paste

I don't know if there is anything cosier than a baked potato. This is my version using a sweet potato for its healthy vibes, sitting comfortably next to my delicious red peppered chicken. I love this meal for its simplicity and great flavours.

1. Preheat the oven to 180°C (160°C fan/350°F/Gas 4).
2. Prick the sweet potato with a fork and bake in the oven for 15 minutes. Meanwhile, coat the chicken breast with the olive oil and season with black pepper and the mixed herbs. Place on a baking tray in the oven with the sweet potato and cook both for a further 25 minutes or until thoroughly cooked through.
3. While they are cooking, make the roasted pepper sauce. Put the roughly chopped red pepper and red onion and place on a baking tray with the garlic clove. Cook in the oven for 15 minutes then remove and add to a blender with the olives, basil, and tomato paste and blitz to a creamy consistency. Add a splash of water if it is too thick.
4. Take the potato and chicken out of the oven and serve on a plate. Cut the potato lengthways and squeeze, then top with the cottage cheese or Greek yogurt.
5. Add the chicken breast and top with the red pepper sauce.
6. Serve with a leafy salad, a wedge of lemon and garnish with fresh basil, if you wish.

GOOD TO KNOW

Be cautious when removing the lid from the blender containing hot food liquid as it can splash and burn your skin

CURRIED COTTAGE PIE

SERVES TWO

- ¾ of a handful of parsnip, peeled and chopped
- ¾ of a handful of swede (rutabaga), peeled and chopped
- 2 tsp coconut oil
- ½ small red onion
- 2 garlic cloves, crushed
- 1 tsp grated fresh ginger root
- lean turkey mince (ground turkey), 2 x the size and thickness of your palm
- 1 tsp garam masala
- ½ tsp ground cumin
- ½ tsp ground coriander
- ½ tsp turmeric
- 1 tbsp tomato paste
- ½ fresh green chilli, finely chopped, plus a couple of slices to garnish
- 200g (7oz) canned chopped tomatoes

A twist on a British classic, the combination of spicy flavours really makes this dish come to life. Using root vegetables for the topping gives it an earthy comforting feel – perfect for warming you up on a cold winter's night.

1. Preheat the oven to 180°C (160°C fan/350°F/Gas 4).
2. First prepare the vegetable topping. Bring a pan of water to the boil and cook the parsnip and swede for around 20 minutes or until soft. Drain, then mash thoroughly until smooth and set aside covered with foil to keep warm.
3. Meanwhile, heat the coconut oil in a non-stick frying pan and gently fry the onion, garlic, and ginger until soft.
4. Add the turkey mince to the pan and continue to cook on a low heat until the mince has turned brown.
5. Add the spices, tomato paste, green chilli, 150ml (⅔ cup) water, and tomatoes and stir well. Cover and simmer on a low heat for 10 minutes.
6. Transfer the mince mixture to an ovenproof dish, then cover with the mashed vegetable topping. Sprinkle a pinch of garam masala over the top and cook in the oven for 10–15 minutes until golden brown on top.
7. If you like a bit of extra heat you can top the finished pie with a couple of slices of green chilli before serving.

CHICKEN AND MUSHROOM PHO

SERVES ONE

- 1 tsp sesame oil
- 1 chicken breast, the size and thickness of your palm, cut into cubes
- 1 garlic clove, chopped
- ¼ courgette (zucchini), spiralized
- 2 chestnut mushrooms, sliced
- small handful of beansprouts
- fresh coriander (cilantro) leaves to garnish

FOR THE STOCK

- 2 handfuls of dried mushrooms
- ½ fresh red chilli, deseeded
- 2 garlic cloves
- 3 lime leaves
- 1 heaped tsp fresh, sliced ginger root
- 3 lime leaves

Experience the perfect pick-me-up with our twist on the traditional Vietnamese noodle soup, pho (pronounced "fuh"). Renowned for its rich and aromatic broth and vibrant herb mix, our version features earthy mushrooms, crunchy bean sprouts, ginger, and garlic – ideal for aiding digestion and reducing nausea and inflammation.

1. In a pan, add all the stock ingredients and 500ml (generous 2 cups) of water, bring to the boil, then turn the heat down, and simmer for 20 minutes.
2. Strain the stock, return the liquid to the pan, then set aside.
3. Meanwhile, heat the oil in a non-stick frying pan over a medium heat. Add the chicken and garlic and fry for 8–10 minutes until cooked through.
4. Now add the vegetables and cook for further 3 minutes.
5. Place the pan of stock over a high heat and bring it back to the boil.
6. To serve, put the chicken and vegetable mix in a bowl, pour over the hot stock, and garnish with coriander leaves.

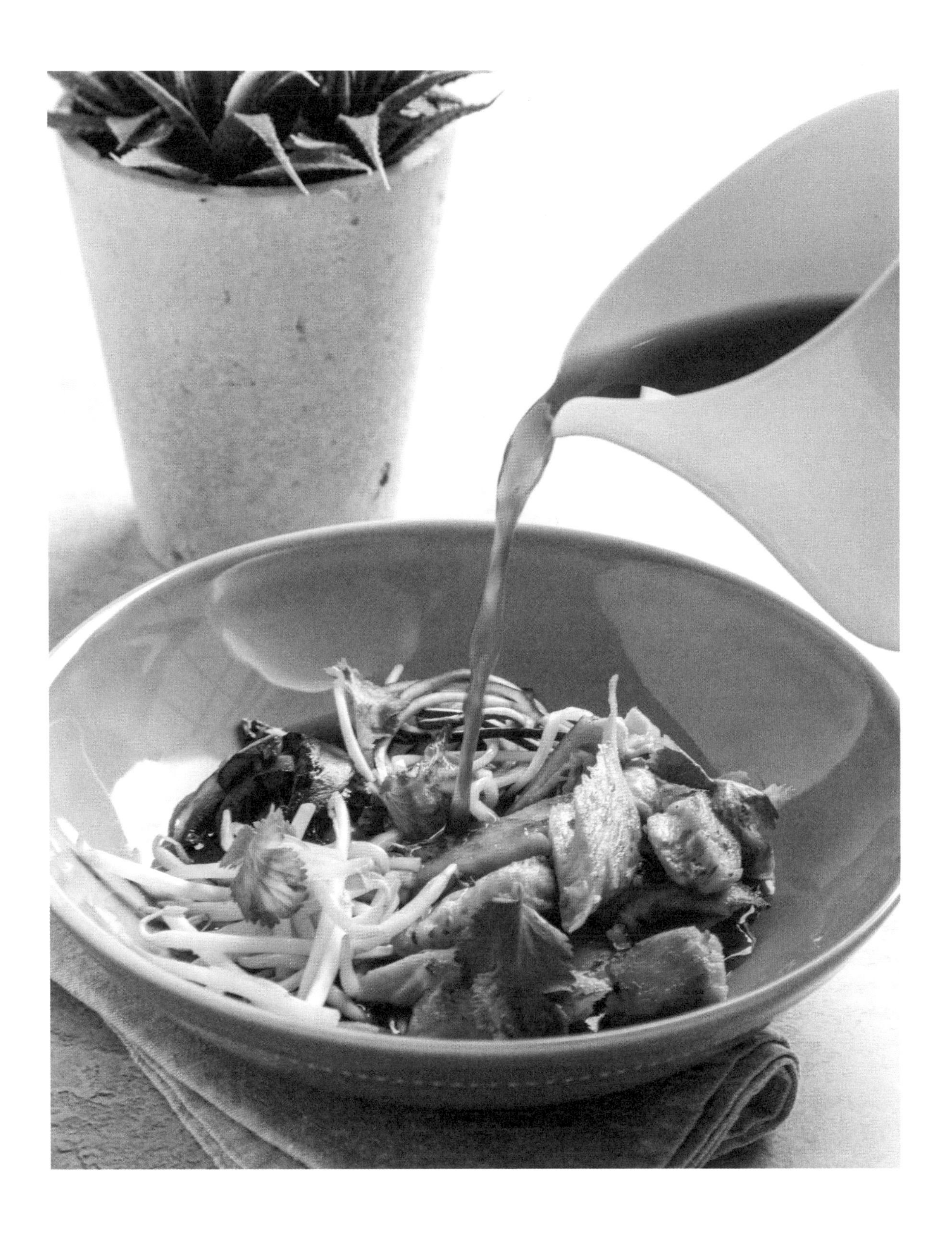

PARSLEY AND LEMON SKATE WITH PEA MASH

SERVES ONE

- 1 skate wing, the size and thickness of your palm
- 1 tsp extra virgin olive oil
- heaped tbsp fresh chopped flat-leaf parsley, plus a little extra to garnish
- 1 lemon – ½ zest, ½ juiced, reserve a wedge for serving
- freshly ground black pepper
- handful of sweet potato, peeled and chopped
- small handful of frozen peas

FOR THE PLANT-BASED GARLIC MAYONNAISE

- 300g (10oz) soft, silken tofu
- 1–2 garlic cloves, crushed
- ½ tsp mustard powder
- squeeze of lemon juice
- splash of unsweetened soya (soy) milk or unsweetened pea milk

Treat yourself to a restaurant-quality meal and elevate your home-dining with my exquisite parsley and lemon skate. It's good enough to grace any fine dining menu when paired with our healthy take on pea mash. Sweet potatoes are packed with more fibre, vitamins, and minerals than white potatoes, making them a more nutrient-dense option.

1. Coat the skate in the olive oil, most of the parsley, the lemon zest, lemon juice, and season with black pepper.
2. Bring a pot of water to the boil and cook the sweet potato for 15–20 minutes until soft and ready to mash.
3. Heat the grill (broiler) to medium. Transfer the fish to a baking tray and grill for 10–15 minutes, turning over halfway. Make sure it is cooked through, then remove from the grill.
4. While the fish is grilling, bring a small pan of water to the boil and cook the peas for a few minutes, drain, then add them to the mashed potato and fold in.
5. Prepare the mayonnaise by putting all the ingredients into the blender and blitzing. Transfer it to a small serving bowl.
6. Finally, garnish the fish with the remaining chopped parsley and season again with black pepper if you wish. Serve with a tablespoon of vegan garlic mayonnaise, the pea mash, and a wedge of lemon.

GOOD TO KNOW

Put the remaining mayonnaise in an airtight container and it will last in the fridge for a few days or, alternatively, you can freeze it in a couple of separate freezer bags and it will last a month.

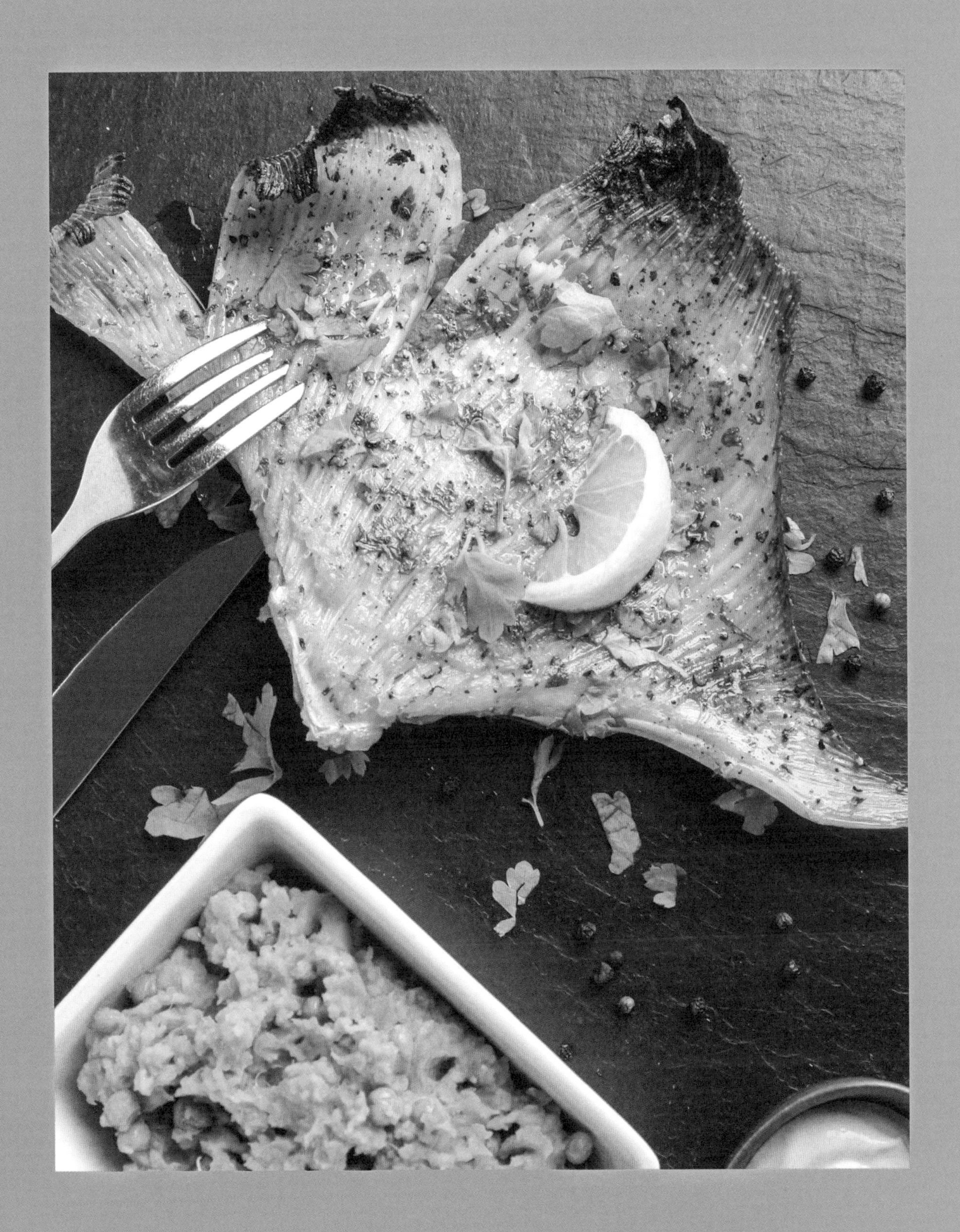

CHICKPEA BIRYANI

SERVES ONE

- 30g (1oz) dry bulgur wheat (90g cooked weight)
- 1 tsp coconut oil
- ½ red onion, finely chopped
- 1 garlic clove, crushed
- 1 tsp grated fresh ginger root
- 400g (14oz) can of chickpeas, drained and rinsed
- 1 tsp curry powder
- ¼ tsp cinnamon
- 200g (7oz) canned chopped tomatoes
- 1 tbsp fresh, chopped coriander (cilantro)
- ½ mango, cut into cubes
- generous squeeze of lime juice

Boss your curry with this super healthy non-traditional biryani recipe. Swapping out traditional rice with bulgur wheat is the key to making this dish shout protein and fibre. Plus, it's perfect for a "fakeaway" Friday night dish.

1. Bring a pan of water to the boil and cook according to the packet instructions (approximately 20 minutes), then drain and set aside.
2. Meanwhile, warm the coconut oil in a non-stick frying pan and fry the red onion for 5 minutes, then add the garlic and ginger and cook for a further 2 minutes. Add the chickpeas, curry powder, cinnamon, canned tomatoes, and coriander. Simmer for 5 minutes until the chickpeas are tender. Take the pan off the heat.
3. Stir the mango through the chickpea mixture, add the cooked bulgur wheat, and mix well.
4. Add the lime juice and serve in your favourite bowl.

GOOD TO KNOW

If you like punchy spicy flavours then choose a hot curry powder but remember to taste test and do not double up on this spice if you are making the recipe for more than one person.

PAD KRAPOW WITH CAULIFLOWER RICE

SERVES ONE

- handful of cauliflower florets
- 1 tsp sesame oil
- Quorn mince (grounds), 1½ x the size and thickness of your palm
- ½ small red onion, finely chopped
- small thumb-size piece fresh ginger root, grated
- ½ red chilli, finely sliced
- 2 lime leaves, finely chopped
- 2 garlic cloves, finely chopped
- juice and zest of 1 lime
- small handful of fresh, chopped Thai basil leaves, plus a few leaves for garnish

In Thailand, "pad" (to stir fry) "krapow" (holy basil, or tulsi), is viewed as a fast-food staple, something to enjoy for a quick lunch. Cauliflower rice is lower in calories and carbohydrates than traditional rice, while providing more fibre and a variety of nutrients. My vegan version of this dish combines all the same flavours and is super speedy, simply perfect for busy on-the-go people.

1. To make the cauliflower rice, grate the cauliflower florets into rice-sized pieces using a box grater.

2. Pour 200ml (scant 1 cup) of water into a non-stick frying pan with the cauliflower rice. Bring to the boil, then reduce the heat and cook over a medium heat for 1 minute. Strain the "rice", transfer it to a mixing bowl, then cover with foil and set aside to keep warm.

3. Meanwhile, add the oil to the non-stick frying pan over a high heat then add the Quorn mince and stir fry for 2 minutes. Next, add the onion, ginger, chilli, lime leaves, and garlic and continue to stir-fry for a further 5 minutes until the onion is soft.

4. Add the lime juice, zest, and fresh basil, stir thoroughly, and remove from the heat. To serve, spoon the cauliflower rice onto a plate and cover with the spicy Thai basil Quorn mince. Garnish with the remaining fresh basil leaves.

MOROCCAN SPICED CAULIFLOWER

SERVES ONE

- 1 large cauliflower "steak"
- 1 tsp extra virgin olive oil
- 1 tsp ground cumin
- 1 tsp cinnamon
- ½ tsp paprika
- 1 tsp sumac
- ½ tsp ground white pepper
- 1 tbsp full-fat Greek yogurt OR Greek-style soya-based vegan yogurt
- 400g (14oz) can of green lentils
- ½ small red onion, finely chopped
- small handful of fresh, finely chopped coriander (cilantro)
- small handful of fresh, finely chopped mint
- small handful of fresh, finely chopped basil
- juice and zest of 1 lime
- 2 tbsp pomegranate seeds

Cauliflower is great for slicing into thick "steaks". The "steaks" readily absorb the flavour of any marinade, and are delicious either roasted or grilled. They are also fat-free, cholesterol-free, and guilt-free, so enjoy!

1. Preheat the oven to 200°C (180°C fan/400°F/Gas 6).
2. Place the cauliflower "steak" in a mixing bowl, drizzle over the olive oil, and sprinkle over the spices. Add the yogurt and turn the cauliflower in the marinade until it is thoroughly coated.
3. Transfer the "steak" onto a non-stick baking tray and cook in the oven for 25 minutes until golden brown.
4. Meanwhile, place the lentils in the same mixing bowl with the onion and chopped herbs and mix with the lime juice, zest, and pomegranate seeds.
5. Serve the "steak" on a plate and spoon the tangy, herby lentil salad on top.

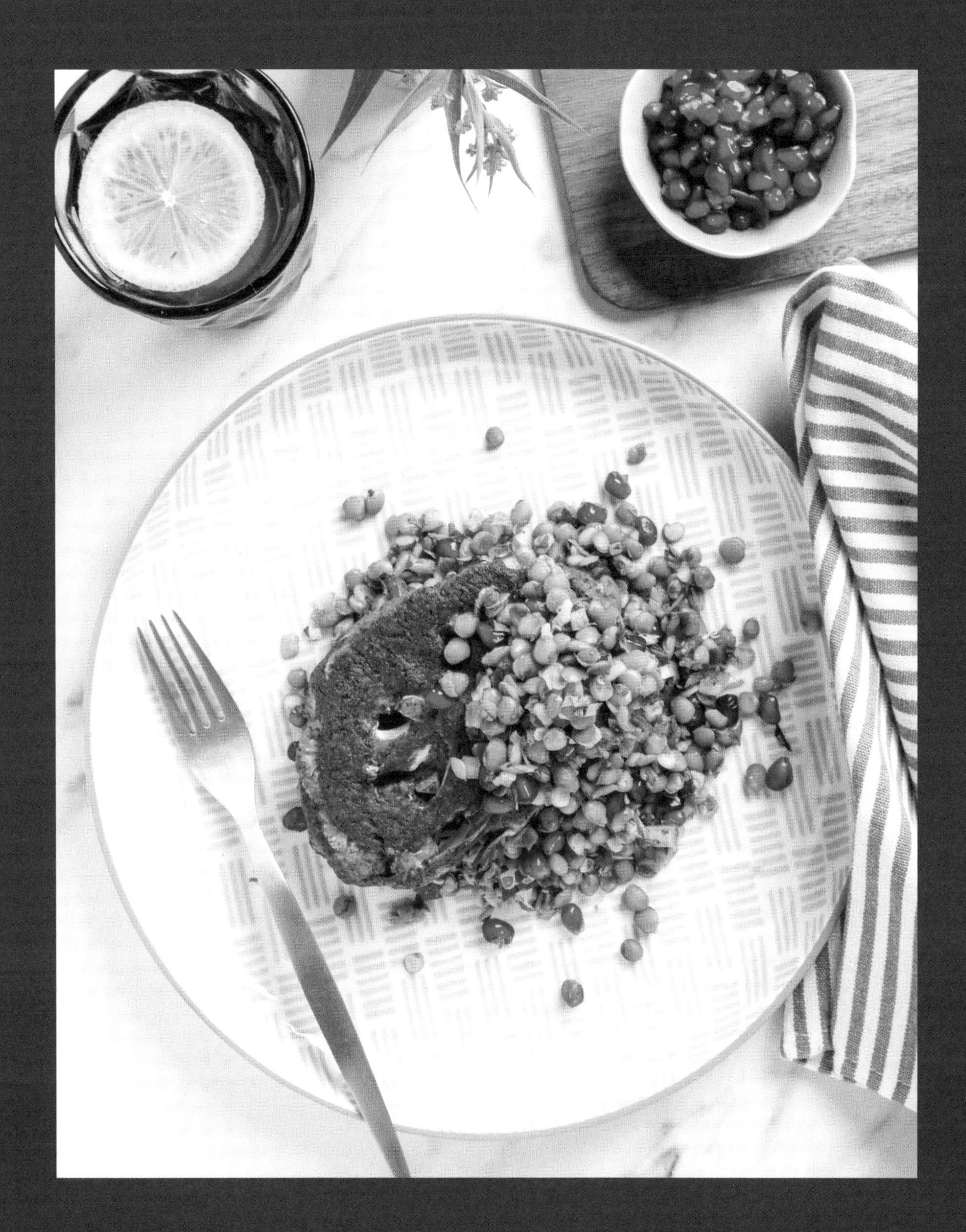

THAI SEA BASS

SERVES ONE

- 1 lemongrass stalk, bashed to release its flavour
- 1 tsp fresh, chopped coriander (cilantro), plus a little extra for garnish
- 1 tsp grated fresh ginger root
- 2 garlic cloves, crushed
- 1 fresh red chilli finely chopped (deseeded if you do not like it too hot)
- zest and juice of ½ lime (reserve ½ to serve)
- 1 tsp extra virgin olive oil
- sea bass fillet, the size and thickness of your palm
- freshly ground black pepper
- handful of sweet potato, chopped into large cubes

This Thai-inspired fish dish is truly sensational. The best bit is when you unwrap a parcel of sea bass infused with Thai flavours. The secret is all in the preparation, the oven takes care of the rest.

1. Preheat the oven to 180°C (160°C fan/350°F/Gas 4).
2. Begin by infusing the fish with Thai spices. Mix the bashed lemongrass with the coriander, ginger, garlic, chilli, the zest and juice of half the lime, and the olive oil.
3. Take a large piece of greaseproof paper and place on a non-stick baking tray. Place the sea bass on the paper, cover it with the Thai spice mixture and season with black pepper.
4. Fold the greaseproof paper around the fish, scrunching it together and sealing it like a closed bag. Cook for 15–20 minutes, depending on the size of the fish.
5. Meanwhile, bring a pot of water to the boil and cook the sweet potato for 15 minutes until soft but not mushy. If you like your sweet potatoes a little brown then cook in a dry, non-stick frying pan over a high heat for a minute or two.
6. Serve the sea bass in its paper with the sweet potatoes on the side with the remaining half a lime.

GOOD TO KNOW

If you're buying a whole sea bass ask your fishmonger to prepare it for you. You can cook this as a whole fish or as fillets.

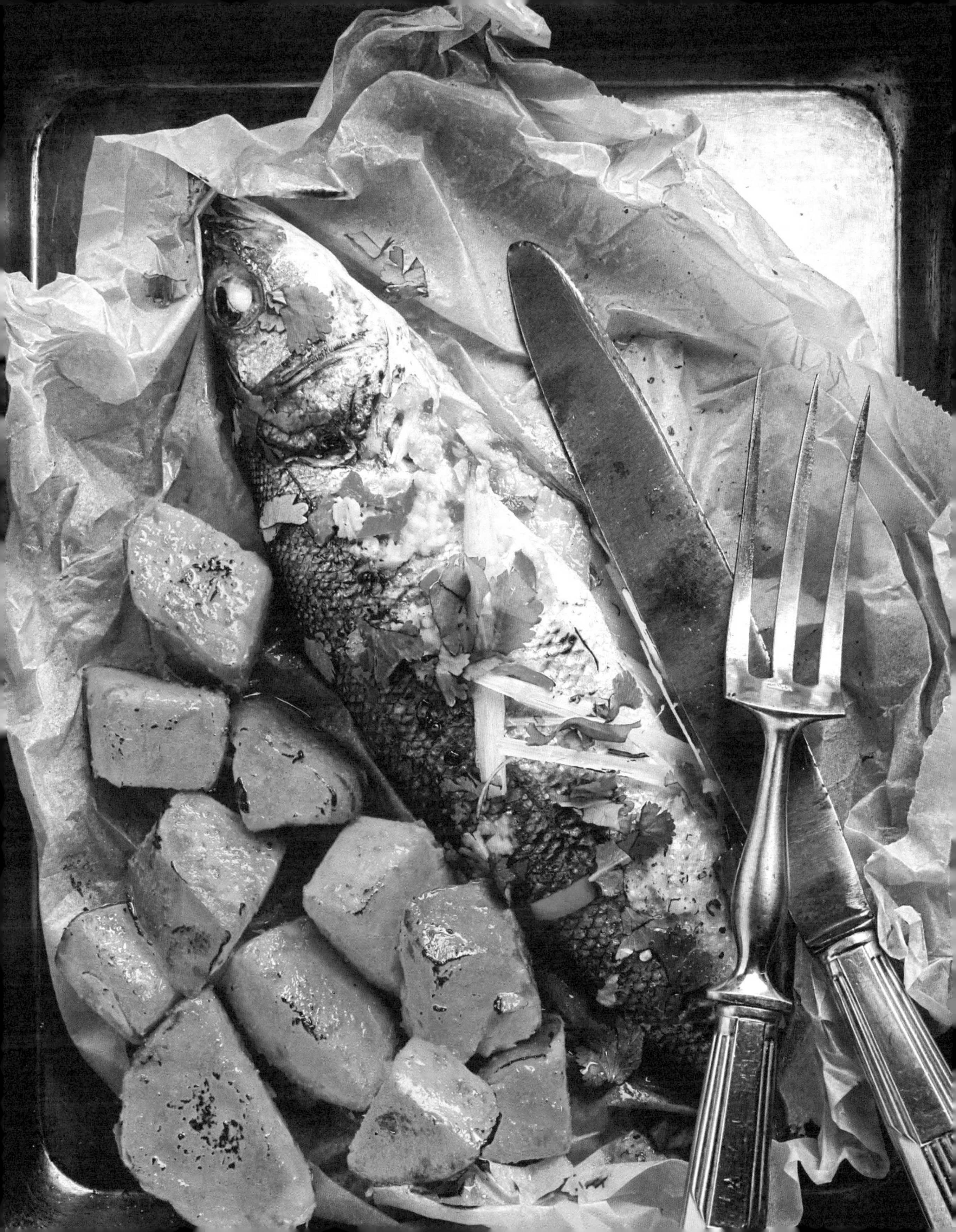

TEMPEH TANDOORI

SERVES TWO

- tempeh, 3 x the size and thickness of your palm, cut into small cubes
- juice of ½ lime
- ½ red onion, chopped
- 1 tbsp full-fat Greek yogurt OR Greek-style soya-(soy-)based vegan yogurt
- 1 tsp grated fresh ginger root
- ½ tsp curry powder
- ½ tsp chilli powder (heat of your choice)
- ½ tsp turmeric
- 4 curry leaves, crumbled
- pinch of ground white pepper
- 2 tsp coconut oil
- 1 cinnamon stick
- 6 cardamom pods, bashed
- 6 cloves
- 2 garlic cloves, crushed
- 1 tsp tomato paste
- 400g (14oz) can of chopped tomatoes
- small handful of fresh, chopped coriander (cilantro), reserving some for garnish
- 80g (⅓ cup) bulgur wheat dry weight (230g/1 cup cooked weight)

Tomatoes, the game-changer of Indian cuisine since the 16th century. Packed with vitamin C, potassium, folate, and vitamin K, they add a sweet-tart-tangy kick to dishes like my divine tempeh tandoori recipe.

1 In a bowl, mix the tempeh, lime juice, onion, yogurt, ginger, curry powder, chilli powder, turmeric, curry leaves, white pepper and put to one side (it can also be left overnight in the fridge).

2 Now heat the coconut oil in a non-stick pan on a medium heat and add the cinnamon stick, cardamom pods, and cloves.

3 Stir for a couple of minutes to release the flavours, then add the garlic, tomato paste, a good splash of water, and stir for another couple of minutes.

4 Next, stir in the canned tomatoes and fresh coriander. Add the marinated tempeh and mix everything together thoroughly. Simmer on a low heat for 20 minutes.

5 Meanwhile, cook the bulgur wheat following the packet instructions.

6 Serve the tandoori and bulgar on your favourite plates, garnished with the remaining coriander.

LENTIL AND MUSHROOM RISOTTO

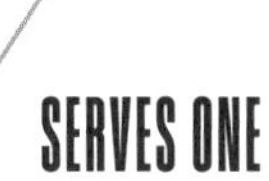

SERVES ONE

1 tsp extra virgin olive oil

¼ stalk celery, thinly sliced

1 shallot, sliced

small handful mushrooms, sliced

1 garlic clove, crushed

4 sprigs fresh sage, stalks removed, leaves chopped

400g (14oz) can of Puy or bijoux lentils, drained and rinsed OR 100g (3½oz) dry Puy lentils

3 cherry tomatoes, quartered

½ handful fresh spinach

freshly ground black pepper

FOR THE TZATZIKI

1 tbsp (14oz) full-fat Greek yogurt OR Greek-style soya-based vegan yogurt

½ cucumber, grated

½ bunch of fresh, chopped mint (stalks removed)

1 sprig fresh, chopped dill

1 or 2 garlic cloves, crushed

½ lemon, squeezed

freshly ground black pepper

Okay, so for all you foodies out there, this isn't risotto as you know it. For a start, it doesn't have a grain of rice in sight. Lentils, however, are one of my favourite superfoods and the perfect option to boost your protein intake. Lentils are naturally gluten free, making them a delicious staple in a gluten-free kitchen.

1 To make the tzatziki, combine all the ingredients in a bowl, finish with ground black pepper to taste. Leave to one side.

2 Gently heat the oil in a large non-stick pan, then add the celery, shallot, mushrooms, garlic, and sage and cook for around 3–5 minutes on a medium heat or until they are just starting to soften.

3 Now add the lentils and tomatoes and cook until warmed through.

4 Add the spinach and cook until slightly wilted.

5 Season with ground black pepper, top with a tablespoon of tzatziki, and serve.

GOOD TO KNOW

I recommend marinating the vegan chicken overnight in the fridge, or for at least 2 hours!

ROASTED MOROCCAN AUBERGINE

SERVES ONE

- ½ small aubergine (eggplant)
- 400g (14oz) can of chickpeas, drained and rinsed (reserve a few whole for garnish)
- juice and zest of ½ lemon
- freshly ground black pepper
- 8 fresh mint leaves
- 1 tbsp pomegranate seeds
- 1 tsp sesame seeds

MARINADE FOR AUBERGINE (EGGPLANT)

- 1 tsp ground cumin
- 1 tsp smoked paprika
- 1 tsp ground coriander
- 1 tsp garlic powder
- 1 tsp dried oregano
- juice of ½ lemon
- 1 tsp extra virgin olive oil

TO SERVE

- small handful of mixed salad

My Middle Eastern bake gets the royal touch here! Silky aubergine topped with delicious shiny pomegranate rubies, golden sesame seeds and fresh mint leaves.

1. Preheat the oven to 180°C (160°C fan/350°F/Gas 4).
2. Take the aubergine and score with a knife diagonally both ways to create a criss-cross pattern (this is to allow the herbs and spices from the marinade to really get into the flesh).
3. In a bowl, combine all the marinade ingredients and mix well. Once combined, use your hands to massage the marinade all over the aubergine.
4. Place the marinated aubergine on a baking tray and put in the oven for 20 minutes.
5. While the aubergine is roasting, add the chickpeas to a blender with the lemon juice and zest and season with a good grind of black pepper. Blitz to a hummus-like consistency.
6. Spread the hummus on a plate, place the roasted aubergine on top, drizzle with olive oil, and garnish with the remaining chickpeas, mint leaves, pomegranate seeds, and sesame seeds. Enjoy with a small side salad.

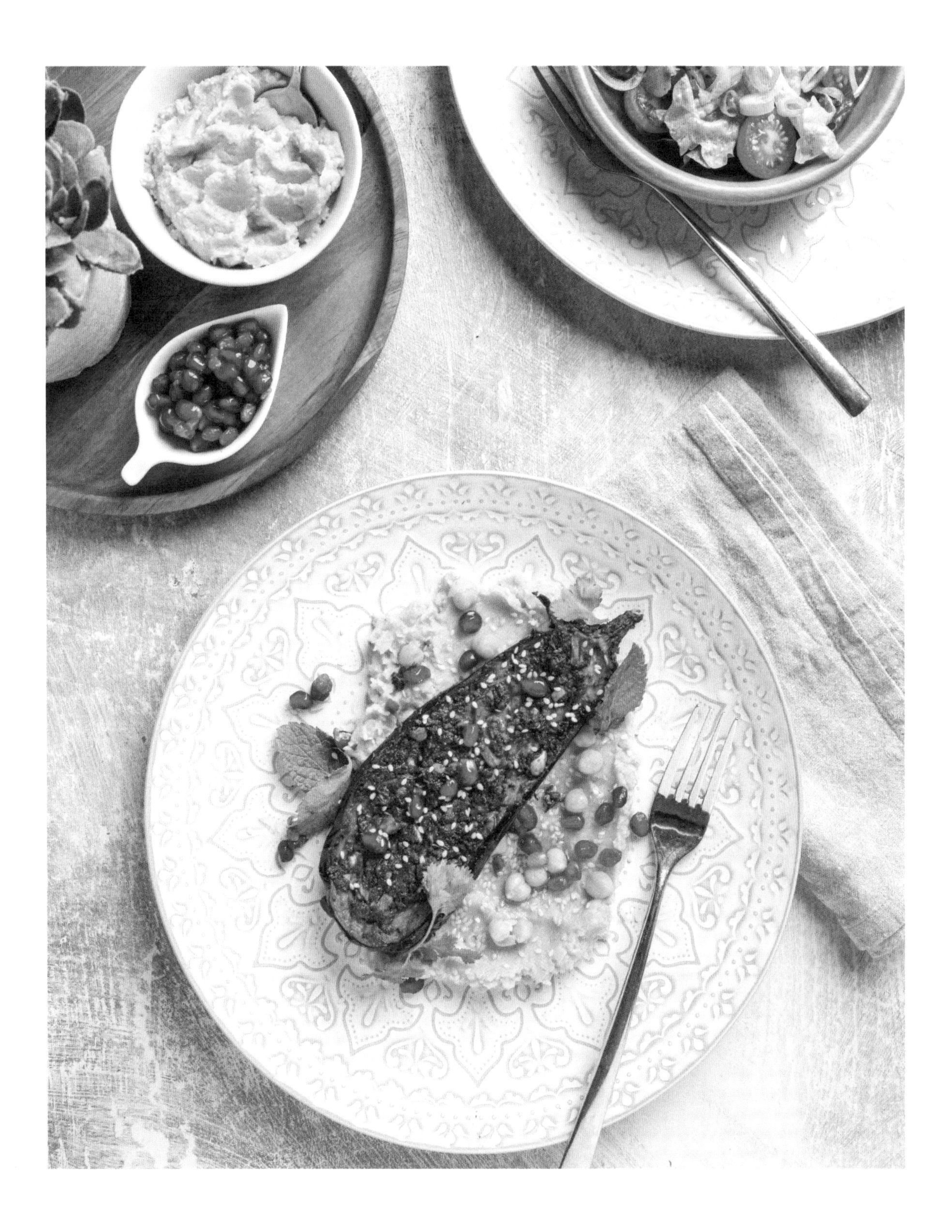

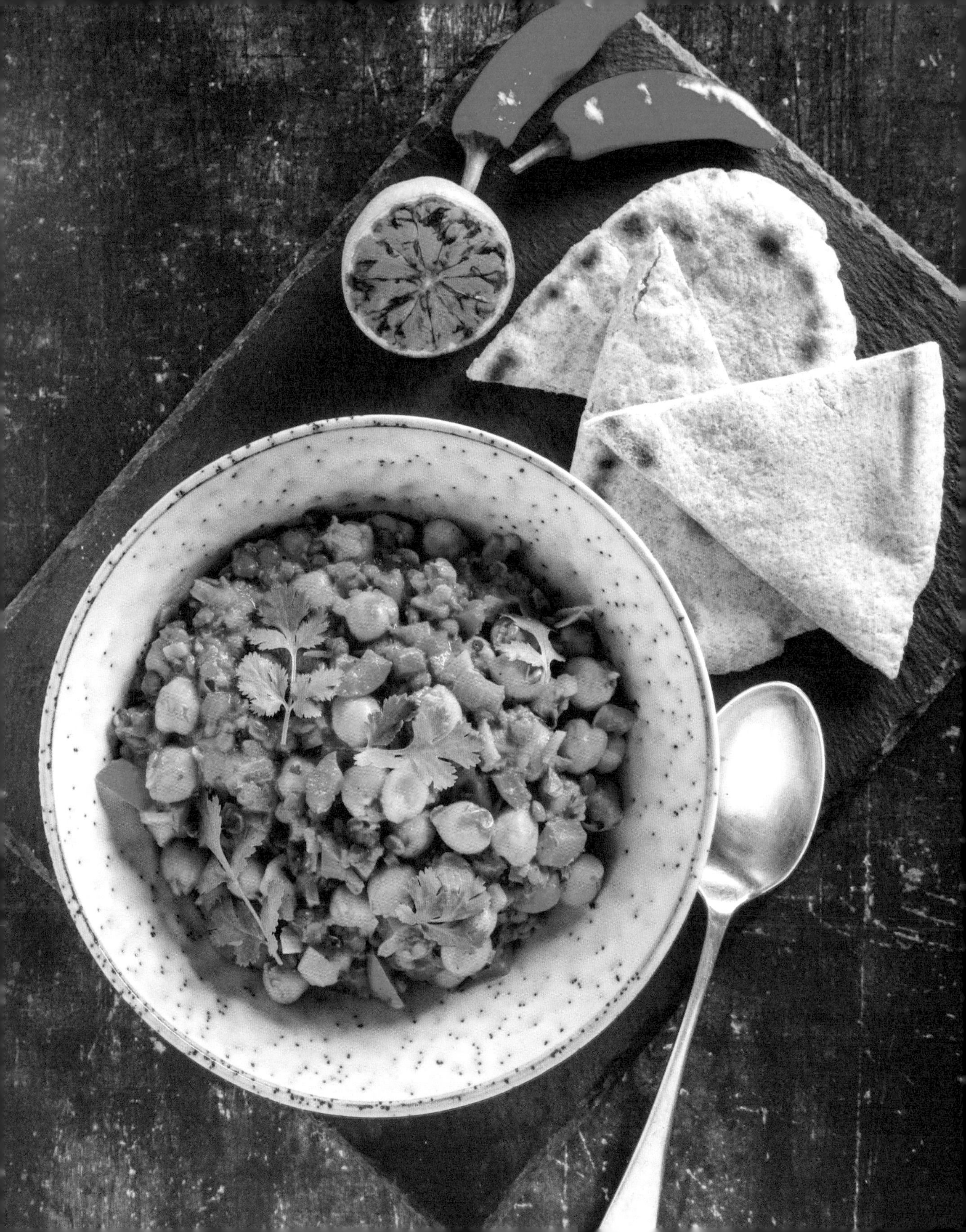

CREAMY LENTIL AND CHICKPEA CURRY

SERVES TWO

- 1 tsp coconut oil
- ½ large white onion, finely chopped
- 1 red pepper, deseeded and diced
- 2 garlic cloves, crushed
- 1 tsp ground cumin
- 1 tsp ground coriander
- 1 tsp turmeric
- 1 tsp garam masala
- 1 tsp curry powder
- ½ tsp chilli powder
- 1 tbsp tomato paste
- 100ml (6½ tbsp) coconut milk
- 400g (14oz) can of chickpeas, drained and rinsed
- 400g (14oz) can of green lentils, drained and rinsed
- small handful of fresh, finely chopped coriander (cilantro), plus a little extra to garnish
- 2 wholemeal pitta breads
- ½ lime

This simple dish is a powerhouse of protein and fibre, supporting digestion and blood sugar control. Who knew the humble yet flavoursome chickpea curry could offer such health benefits?

1. Preheat the oven to 180°C (160°C fan/350°F/Gas 4).
2. Heat the oil in a non-stick pan over a low to medium heat, add the onion, pepper, and garlic and cook until softened.
3. Add the spices and stir so that they completely coat the onion, pepper, and garlic.
4. Add the tomato paste, coconut milk, 200ml (scant 1 cup) of water, and the chickpeas to the pan and bring to the boil. Then turn down the heat and add the green lentils and chopped coriander and let simmer for 10 minutes.
5. Pop the pittas in the oven for 2 minutes before serving to warm through.
6. Divide the curry between two bowls, garnish with some fresh coriander and a good squeeze of lime. Serve with the warm pitta.

LIME AND PEPPER SWORDFISH WITH POTATO SALAD

SERVES ONE

swordfish, the size and thickness of your palm

1 tsp extra virgin olive oil

juice and zest of 1 lime (reserve a wedge to garnish)

freshly ground black pepper

FOR THE POTATO SALAD

1 handful of sweet potato, chopped into cubes

½ tbsp full-fat Greek yogurt OR Greek-style soya-based vegan yogurt

½ spring onion, finely sliced

1 tsp fresh, chopped coriander (cilantro), plus a little extra to garnish

1 tsp chopped flat-leaf parsley

freshly ground black pepper

TO SERVE

small handful of salad leaves

Sometimes the simplest meals are the best and this is no exception. This meaty fish, packed with an abundance of nutrients, when combined with the zingy lime and the herby sweet potato salad makes the perfect meal.

1. To make the potato salad, boil the sweet potato for approximately 15 minutes or until cooked through, then drain and leave to cool. When cooled, mix with the remaining ingredients in a bowl, season with black pepper, and garnish with coriander.

2. Coat the swordfish in the olive oil, lime juice, and zest.

3. Season the fish generously with black pepper and grill (broil) or griddle for approximately 6 minutes on each side or until cooked through.

4. Serve on a plate with the salad leaves, potato salad, and a wedge of lime.

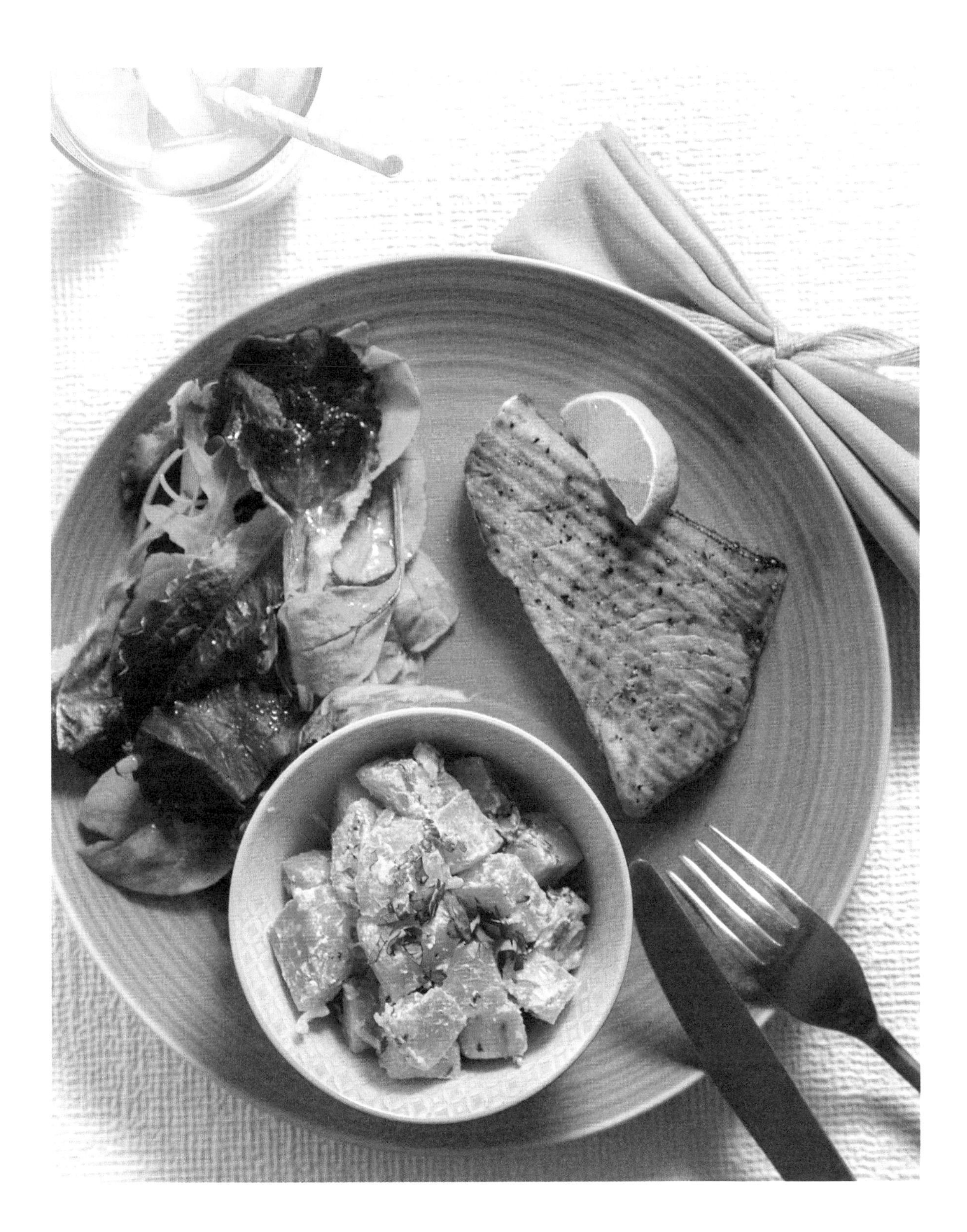

PAD THAI

SERVES ONE

- small handful of courgette (zucchini)
- ½ tsp sesame oil
- 1 chicken breast, the size and thickness of your palm, cut into cubes
- ½ handful of red pepper, deseeded and sliced
- ½ fresh chilli, finely chopped
- 1 garlic clove, peeled and crushed
- 1 tsp grated fresh ginger root
- 1 spring (green) onion, sliced
- ½ lime

TO SERVE

- 3 almonds, chopped
- few sprigs of fresh, chopped coriander (cilantro)

Pad Thai has become a bit of a modern classic and particularly popular within "street food" culture. I wanted to replicate the Thai flavours by including spring onion, zesty lime, and fresh ginger for my version without all the added and unnecessary salt and sugar.

1. Prepare a handful of courgette ribbons by slicing with a potato peeler lengthways.
2. Heat the sesame oil in a non-stick frying pan and add the chicken, pepper, chilli, garlic, ginger, and sliced spring onion then fry quickly over a medium to high heat, stirring continually for 4 minutes.
3. Next, add the courgette ribbons and a squeeze of lime.
4. Stir-fry for a couple of minutes or until the courgette just starts to soften and your chicken is cooked through.
5. Serve in a bowl and garnish with the almonds and coriander.

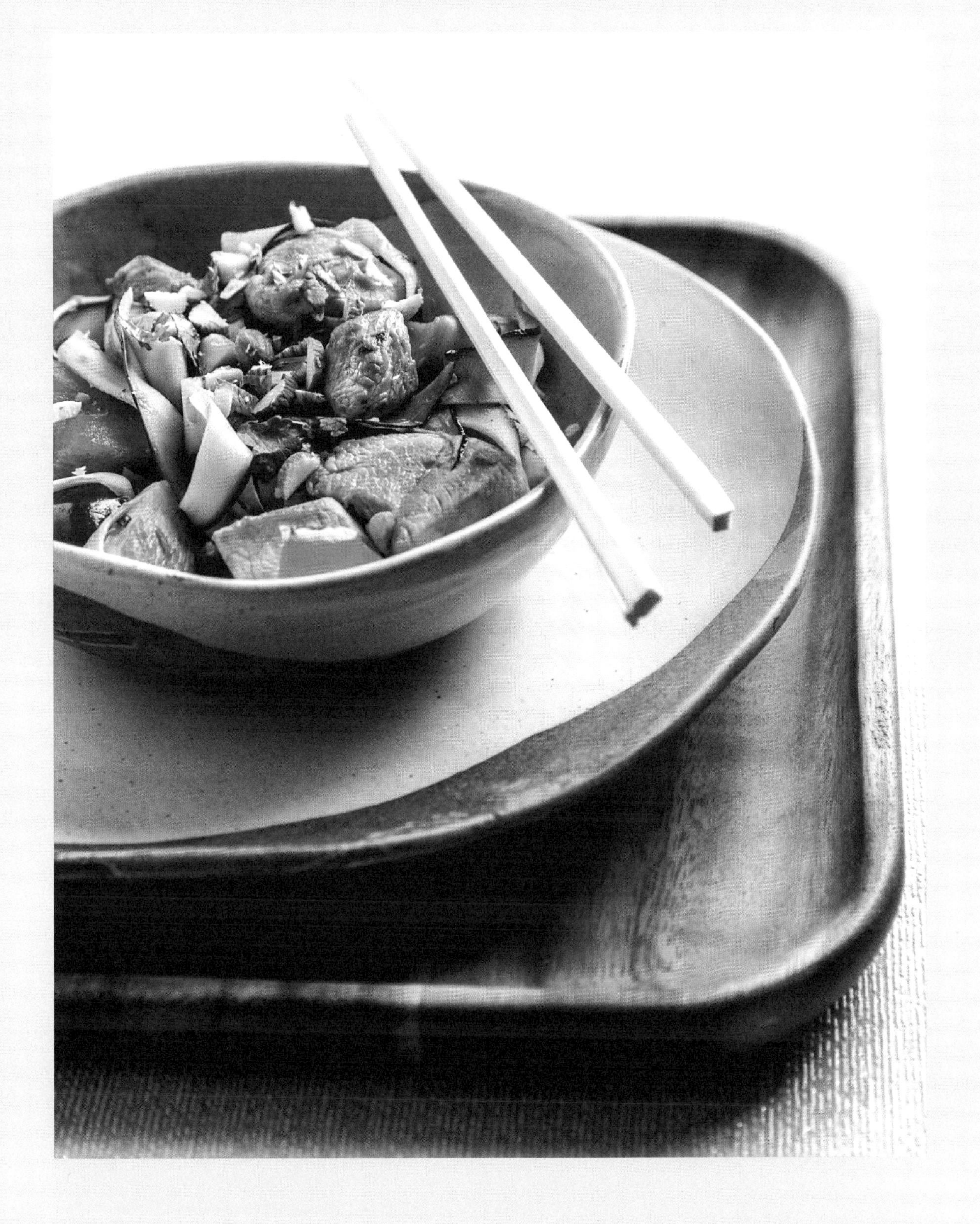

CHICKPEA TAGINE

SERVES TWO

- 1 tsp extra virgin olive oil
- ½ red onion, roughly chopped
- 3 garlic cloves, finely chopped
- 1 tsp turmeric
- 1 tsp ground ginger
- 1 tsp chilli flakes (optional)
- large combined handful of a mixture of red, green, or yellow peppers, courgette (zucchini), and aubergine (eggplant), roughly chopped
- 2 x 400g (14oz) cans of chickpeas, drained and rinsed
- 400g (14oz) can of chopped tomatoes
- small handful of dried apricots, chopped
- 2 tsp flaked almonds
- small handful of fresh, chopped flat-leaf parsley
- small handful of fresh, chopped coriander (cilantro)

Who doesn't love a quick one-pot meal? This one certainly doesn't disappoint. With a nod to Morocco, this stew is ram-packed full of flavour. Plus, the sweetness of the apricots is complemented perfectly by the crunchy toasted almonds.

1. Preheat the oven to 180°C (160°C fan/350°F/Gas 4).
2. Add the olive oil, onion, garlic, spices, and chilli flakes to a pan and fry for 5 minutes over a low to medium heat until softened slightly.
3. Add the peppers, courgette, aubergine, chickpeas, canned tomatoes, and apricots, bring to the boil, then simmer for 15 minutes.
4. Meanwhile, place the almonds on a baking tray and cook in the oven for 2 minutes or until lightly toasted.
5. When the vegetables in the tagine are cooked, add the chopped herbs and stir well.
6. To serve, spoon the tagine into a bowl and garnish with the toasted almonds.

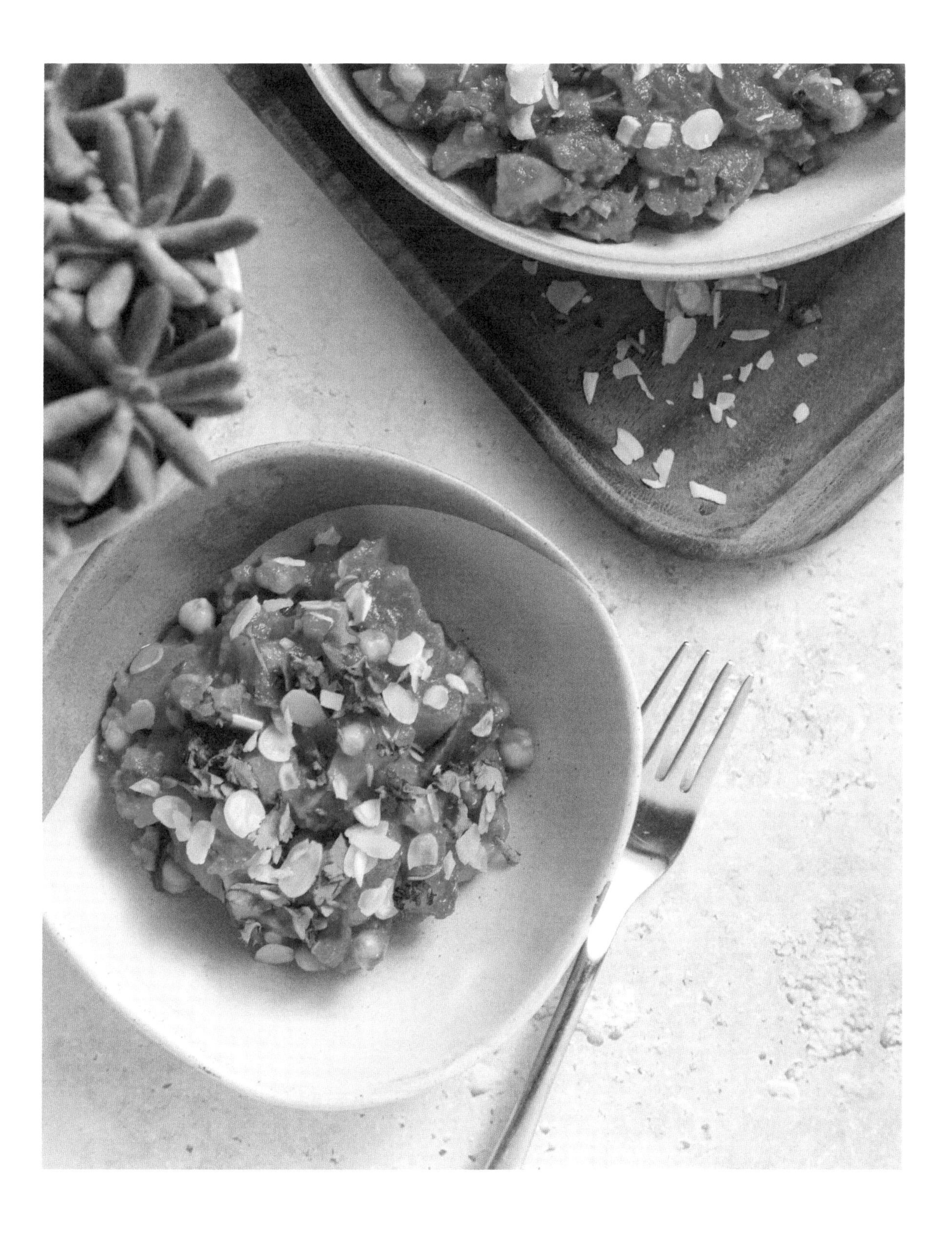

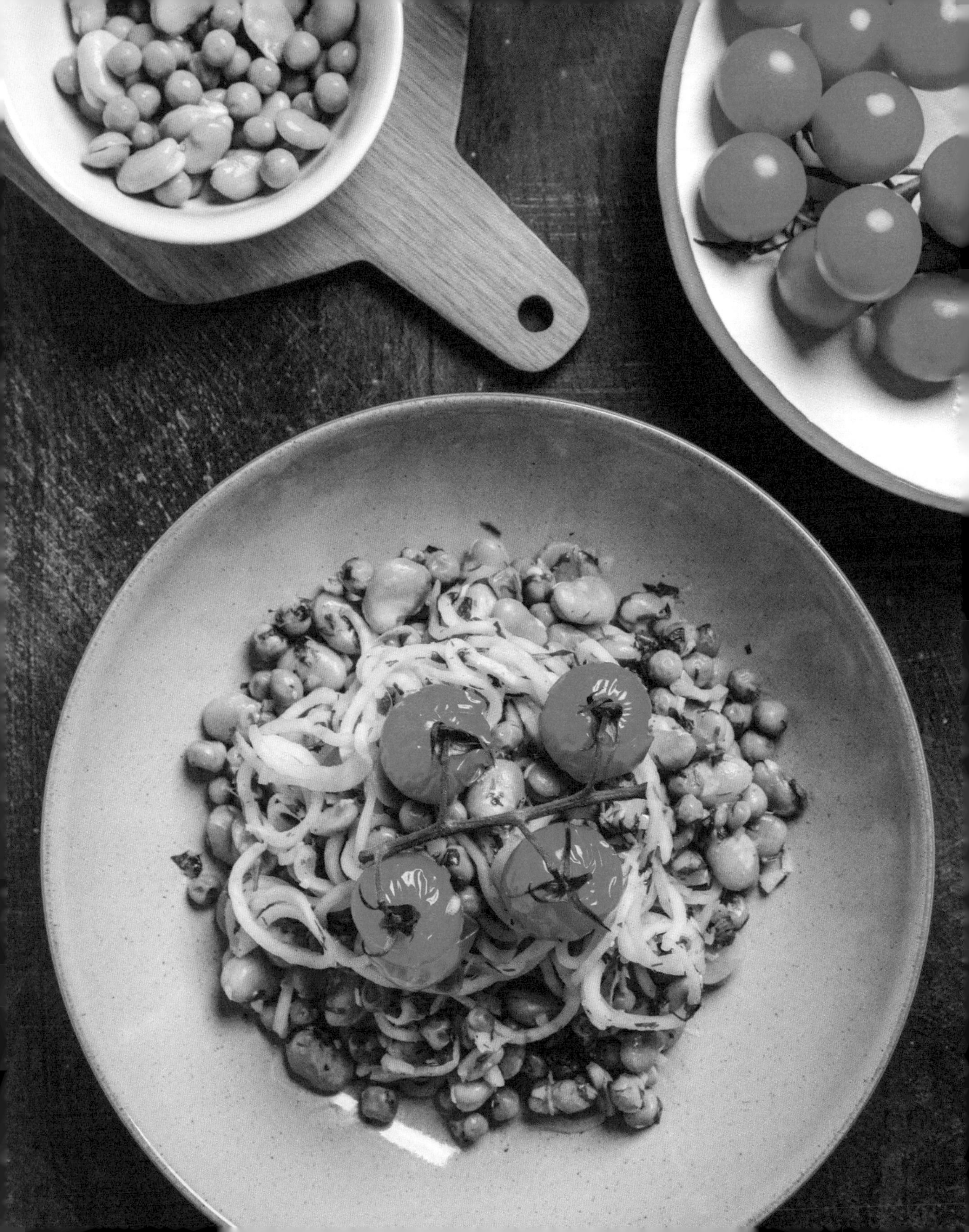

BROAD BEAN AND CELERIAC SINGUINI

SERVES ONE

- small handful of celeriac, peeled
- 4 cherry tomatoes
- 1 tsp extra virgin olive oil
- 1 garlic clove, chopped
- 200g (7oz) broad (fava) beans (fresh or frozen), peeled
- ½ tsp ground white pepper
- small handful of garden peas (fresh or frozen)
- zest and juice of ½ lemon
- handful of chopped fresh herbs (parsley, dill, and mint)

What on earth is singuini? The word "sin" in Spanish means "without", so it is my play on the word "linguine", made using a vegetable and therefore is without pasta! Celeriac has always been the underdog to the potato. However, with its nutty flavour, health benefits and the fantastic invention of the spiralizer, we can enjoy the advantages of improved digestion and bone health with this quick and easy mid-week supper.

1. Preheat the oven to 180°C (160°C fan/350°F/Gas 4).
2. Using a spiralizer, turn the celeriac into "noodles" or use a potato peeler to create ribbons.
3. Place a pan of water over a high heat and bring to the boil. Add the celeriac, cook for 1 minute, then drain and set aside.
4. Meanwhile, put the cherry tomatoes on a baking tray and place in the oven for 5 minutes.
5. In a medium non-stick frying pan, add the olive oil, garlic, and broad beans and fry for 2 minutes over a medium heat, seasoning with white pepper.
6. Now add the peas, lemon zest, and fresh herbs and stir well. Then add the celeriac and lemon juice and combine all the ingredients together.
7. Transfer the celeriac mixture to a pasta dish and serve with the cooked cherry tomatoes on top.

JERK SALMON WITH GRIDDLED VEGETABLES

SERVES ONE

- 1 salmon fillet, the size and thickness of your palm
- 1 tsp dried mixed herbs
- ½ tsp allspice
- ½ tsp cinnamon
- ½ tsp ground white pepper
- 1 tsp extra virgin olive oil
- 4 vine cherry tomatoes
- 5 button (closed cup) mushrooms
- 2 large slices aubergine (eggplant)
- 8 slices courgette (zucchini)

Jerk spices can be used on pretty much any meat or fish. However, I like them best when combined with the full flavour of salmon. This quick and simple recipe is served with a portion of delicious colouful vegetables. Salmon is rich in omega-3 fatty acids, which can help reduce inflammation, improve heart health, and support brain function.

1. Preheat the oven to 180°C (160°C fan/350°F/Gas 4).
2. Put the salmon on a plate. Mix all the spices together and then rub them over the salmon to coat.
3. Transfer the fish to a non-stick baking tray and roast in the oven for 15–20 minutes, or until cooked.
4. Meanwhile, add the olive oil to a griddle or frying pan and cook the vegetables to your liking.
5. Arrange the salmon and vegetables on the plate of your choice and serve.

MEDITERRANEAN COTTAGE PIE WITH LENTILS

SERVES TWO

- large handful sweet potato, peeled and diced
- 1 tsp extra virgin olive oil
- 2 garlic cloves, chopped
- 1 small red onion, diced
- 6 pitted olives (green or black), sliced
- 1 tsp sumac
- 1 tsp paprika
- 400g (14oz) can of chopped tomatoes
- 1 tsp dried basil
- 1 tsp dried oregano
- 1 tsp dried parsley
- 2 x 400g (14oz) cans of Puy lentils, drained and rinsed
- ½ tsp ground white pepper

The ultimate makeover! The British cottage pie has been elevated to new-found heights with the flavours of all things Mediterranean. It's packed with vibrant vegetables, lean protein, and aromatic herbs. Delicioso! Puy lentils are so good – quick to cook and great source of plant-based protein.

1. Preheat the grill to a medium heat.
2. Bring a pot of water to the boil and cook the sweet potatoes for 15–20 minutes until soft enough to mash. Drain, mash, and set aside covered with foil to keep warm.
3. Place a large non-stick saucepan over a low heat. Add the olive oil, garlic, onion, olives, sumac, and paprika and gently fry until the onions are soft.
4. Add the canned tomatoes and herbs to the pan and simmer for 10 minutes.
5. Next, add the cooked lentils and white pepper to the sauce and stir well.
6. Transfer the lentil mixture to a small ovenproof dish and top with the sweet potato mash. Place the dish under the grill until the potato has browned, then serve.

KATSU TOFU BURGER

SERVES 1

- firm tofu, 1½ x the size and thickness of your palm
- 1 tbsp almond milk (enough to cover the tofu when dipping)
- 1 tbsp flaxseeds (enough to cover the tofu when dipping)
- freshly ground black pepper
- 1 wholemeal flatbread
- 1 radish, thinly sliced
- few ribbons of cucumber (I use a potato peeler to slice)
- ½ spring (green) onion, sliced
- small handful of salad leaves

KATSU CURRY SAUCE

- ½ tsp grated fresh ginger root
- 1 garlic clove, crushed
- ½ red onion, finely chopped
- 1 tsp coconut oil
- ½ tsp garam masala
- ½ tsp mild curry powder
- tiny squeeze of lemon juice
- 1 heaped tsp full-fat Greek yogurt OR Greek-style soya-based vegan yogurt

All the flavours of a Japanese curry, in the form of a burger. That's right, I'm mixing it up with a simple twist that whips up a storm, combining the sweet and spice from the katsu with the smooth creaminess of the tofu. Add a bit of crunch with radish, and it is just good food!

1 Preheat the oven to 180°C (160°C fan/350°F/Gas 4).

2 Dip the tofu in the almond milk to cover and then coat with the flaxseed.

3 Season the tofu generously with black pepper, place on a non-stick baking tray and cook on 20–25 minutes, turning halfway through.

4 Meanwhile, prepare the katsu sauce. In a small pan, fry the ginger, garlic, and onion in the coconut oil on a low heat for 5 minutes. Add the garam masala and curry powder and stir. Then add 100ml (6½ tbsp) water, stir, and bring to the boil. Finally, add the lemon juice and yogurt.

5 Transfer the mix to a blender and blitz for 1 minute until it has a sauce-like consistency.

6 When everything is ready, load the flatbread with the tofu burger and the salad. Drizzle over the katsu sauce and serve.

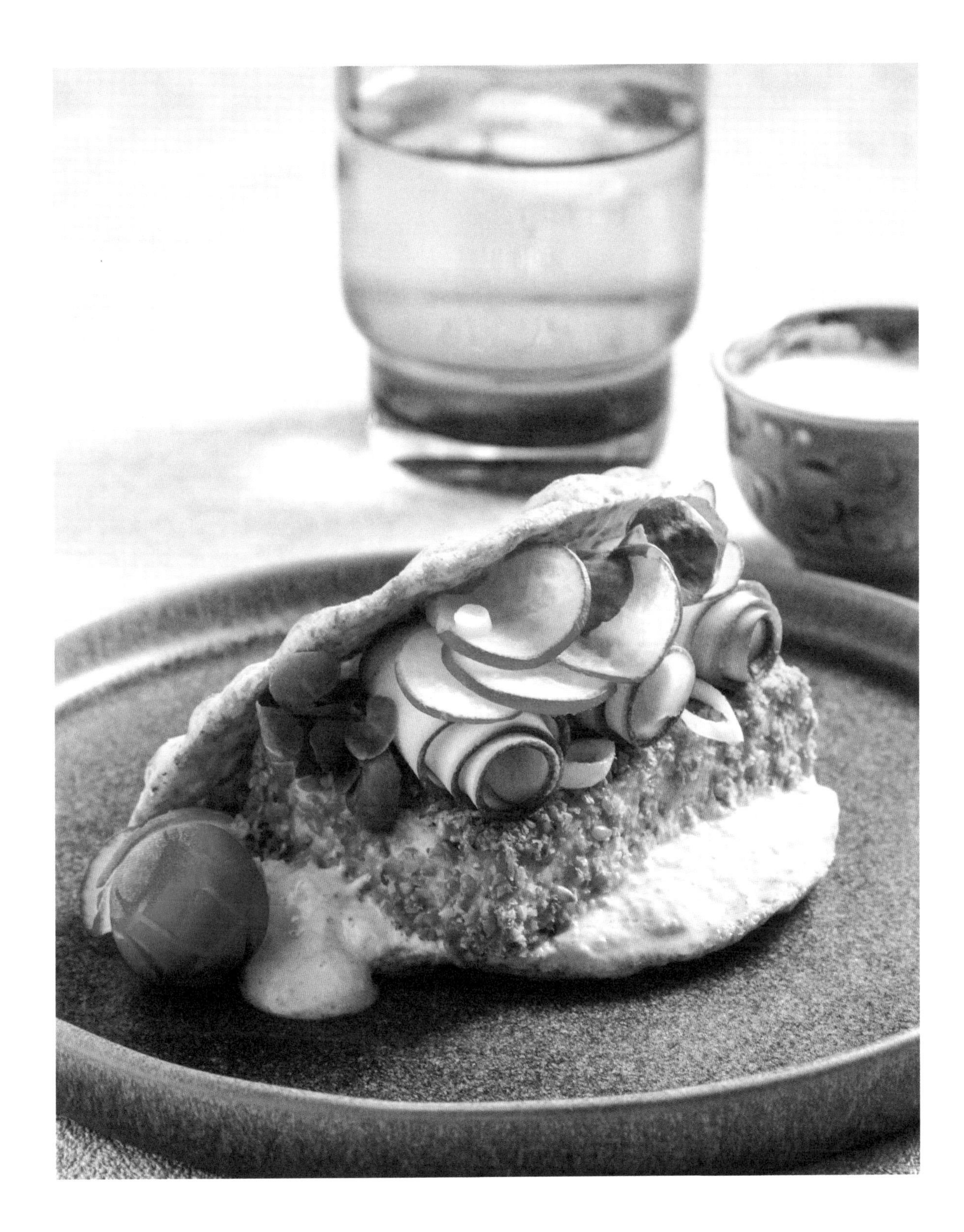

CHICKEN CHOW MEIN WITH CELERIAC NOODLES

SERVES FOUR

- 1 medium-sized celeriac, peeled
- chicken breast, 4 x the size and thickness of your palm, cut into cubes
- 2 tsp sesame oil
- small handful of red or green pepper, deseeded and sliced
- small handful of mushrooms, sliced
- small handful of beansprouts
- small handful of fresh, chopped coriander (cilantro)
- handful of fresh, chopped basil

FOR THE MARINADE

- 1 heaped tsp grated fresh ginger root
- 1 red chilli, finely chopped (deseeded if you do not like it too hot)
- juice and zest of 1 lime
- 2 tsp sesame seeds
- 3 garlic cloves, crushed
- small handful of fresh, chopped coriander (cilantro)
- 1 tsp Chinese five spice

TO SERVE

- 12 cashew nuts, chopped
- 4 lime wedges

Packed with colourful veggies and protein-rich vegan chicken, this guilt-free "fakeaway" will satisfy those weekend cravings while nourishing your body. With celeriac noodles and fresh herbs, it's a healthy feast that's sure to impress your friends at your next gathering!

1. Using a spiralizer, turn the celeriac into "noodles" or use a potato peeler to create ribbons.
2. Make the marinade by combining all the ingredients in a mixing bowl, then add the chicken pieces and mix thoroughly.
3. Heat the oil in a large non-stick frying pan or wok over a high heat, add the marinated chicken pieces and stir fry for 5 minutes. Add the pepper and mushrooms and stir-fry for another 2 minutes.
4. Now add the celeriac noodles, beansprouts and chopped herbs, and stir-fry for a further 3 minutes, making sure the chicken is cooked through.
5. To serve, use a pair of tongs and divide the chow mein equally between four bowls, garnish with a sprinkle of the chopped cashew nuts and a wedge of lime.

PLANT-BASED MINCE KAPUSKA

SERVES TWO

- 1 red pepper, whole
- 1 tsp extra virgin olive oil
- 1 white onion, finely chopped
- 1 garlic clove, crushed
- Quorn mince (grounds) or soya mince (soy crumbles), the size the thickness of your palm
- 2 tomatoes
- 1 tbsp and 1 tsp tomato paste
- ½ tsp chilli flakes
- 1 tsp fennel seeds
- 6 pitted black or green olives, finely sliced
- freshly ground black pepper
- 1 large handful white or Savoy cabbage, shredded
- 4 dried apricots, finely chopped

A meat-free version of the classic Turkish cabbage stew recipe. This is humble old-world comfort food that's also good for you! The addition of fennel seeds and apricots gives this dish a rich, sweet, slightly liquorice-scented flavour.

1 Preheat the oven to 200°C (180°C fan/400°F/Gas 6).

2 Place the whole red pepper on a non-stick baking tray and cook for 20–30 minutes until slightly charred.

3 Take the roasted red pepper out of the oven and leave it to one side to cool.

4 In a non-stick pan, warm the olive oil at a medium heat and gently fry the onion and garlic until the onion is softened and translucent. Add the Quorn or soya mince to the pan and stir-fry gently for 5 minutes.

5 Peel the tomatoes by scoring the skins with a sharp knife, placing them in a small heatproof bowl or large mug and covering with boiling water. Leave the tomatoes for a few minutes, then remove from the water, and the skins should peel off. Roughly chop the tomatoes and then add to the pan along with 1 tablespoon of tomato paste, the chilli flakes, and fennel seeds.

6 Take the cooled red pepper and remove the skin, stalk, and seeds. Place in a food processor with 1 teaspoon of tomato paste and blitz to a paste. Add the pepper paste to the pan, along with the olives.

7 Season with black pepper, then add 350ml (1¼ cups) water to the pan, bring to the boil, throw in the shredded cabbage, and reduce to a low heat. Cover and simmer for 20 minutes until the cabbage is tender.

8 Stir in the chopped apricots and serve in your favourite bowls.

FISH AND CHIPS WITH CHIP SHOP CURRY SAUCE

SERVES ONE

- handful of sweet potato, sliced into chunky chips
- 1 cod fillet (or other white fish), the size and thickness of your palm
- freshly ground black pepper
- small sprig of rosemary, leaves finely chopped

FOR THE CURRY SAUCE

- ½ tsp grated fresh ginger root
- 1 garlic clove, crushed
- ½ red onion, finely chopped
- 1 tsp coconut oil
- ½ tsp garam masala
- ½ tsp mild curry powder
- tiny squeeze of lemon juice
- 1 heaped tsp full-fat Greek yogurt OR Greek-style soya-based vegan yogurt

My simple adaptation of a British favourite. Add in my guilty pleasure of chip shop curry sauce and you have a healthy version of a wonderfully nostalgic recipe.

1. Preheat the oven to 180°C (160°C fan/350°F/Gas 4).
2. Season the fish with black pepper and sprinkle over the chopped rosemary.
3. Put the chips on a baking tray in the oven for 30 minutes.
4. Begin to prepare the curry sauce by adding the coconut oil to a non-stick pan and frying the ginger, garlic, and onion on a low heat for 5 minutes.
5. Now put the fish under the grill (broiler) for 15 minutes. Turn the fish after half the cooking time and shake the chips, so they don't stick.
6. Add the garam masala and curry powder to the curry sauce and continue to stir. Pour in 100ml (6½ tbsp) of water then bring to the boil, reduce the heat, and allow the liquid to reduce, until it reaches a sauce-like consistency.
7. Remove the sauce from the heat, squeeze over the lemon juice and stir in the spoonful of yogurt. Transfer the sauce to a blender and blitz for one minute.
8. Arrange the fish and chips on a plate or wrap them in some baking paper with the sauce in a small dish on the side for dipping.

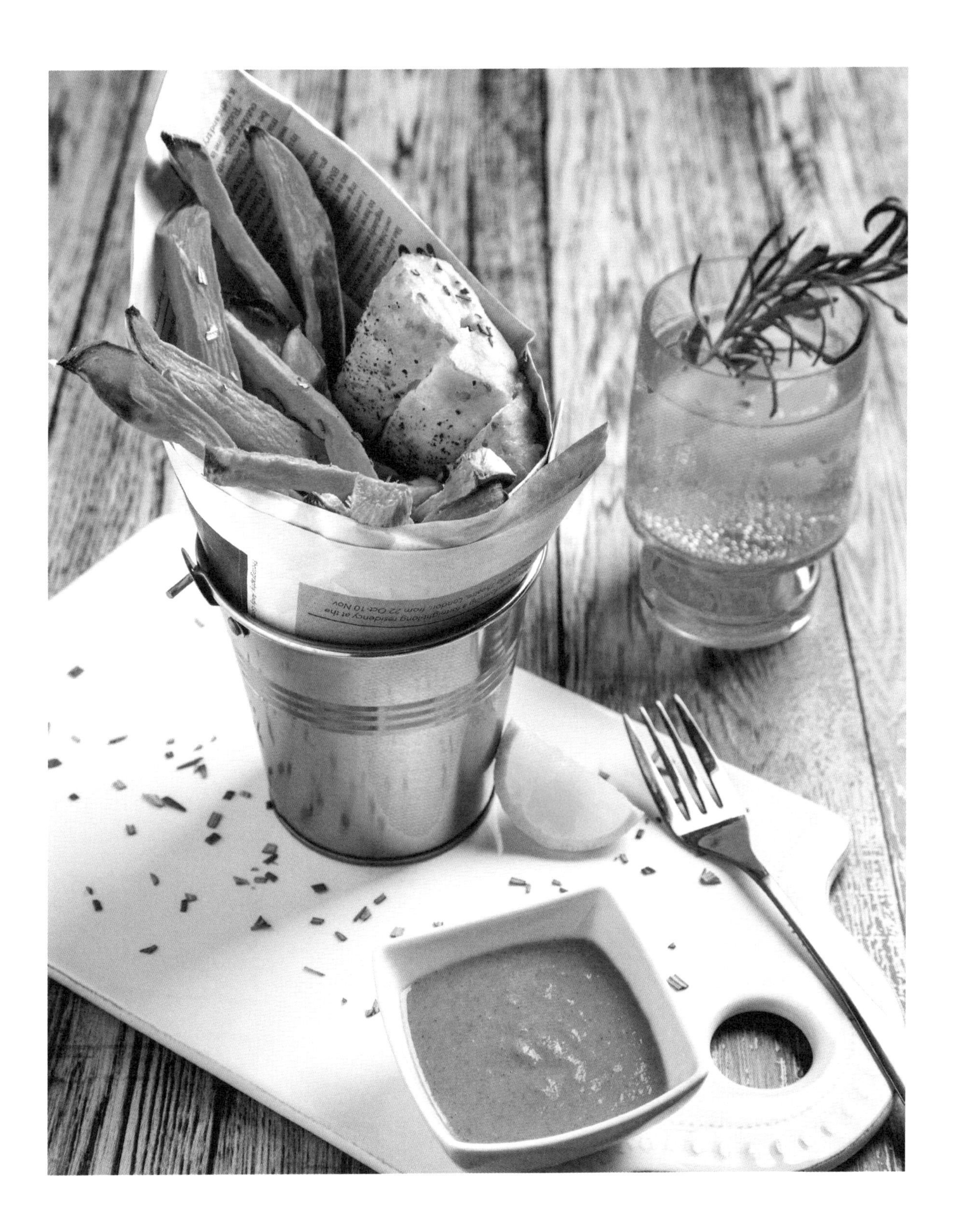

VEGAN ALOO KEEMA

SERVES TWO

- handful of sweet potato, peeled and cut into cubes
- 2 tsp coconut oil
- ½ small red onion, finely chopped
- 2 tsp grated fresh ginger root
- 1 garlic clove, crushed
- 1 fresh green chilli, finely chopped
- Quorn or soya mince, 3 x the size and thickness of your palm
- ½ can (200g) of chopped tomatoes
- 1 tsp garam masala
- 1 tsp ground cumin
- ½ tsp ground coriander
- handful of frozen peas
- 2 tbsp fresh, chopped coriander (cilantro), plus a little extra to garnish

I've given this classic Indian recipe a special vegan makeover. Sweet potato for the aloo enhances the spices and gives this flavourful dish a health kick of vitamins, including vitamins C and B6, which are vital for your brain and nervous system.

1. Bring a pot of water to the boil and cook the sweet potatoes for 15–20 minutes until soft.
2. Meanwhile, place a non-stick pan over a medium heat. Add the onion and fry until softened, then add the ginger, garlic, and chilli and cook on a medium heat for a couple of minutes.
3. Now add the Quorn or soya mince, chopped tomatoes, spices, peas, and a good splash of water, and stir thoroughly. Cook on a medium to low heat for approximately 10 minutes.
4. Add the potatoes and fresh coriander and mix together gently.
5. When it's all piping hot, serve it in your favourite bowls, and enjoy.

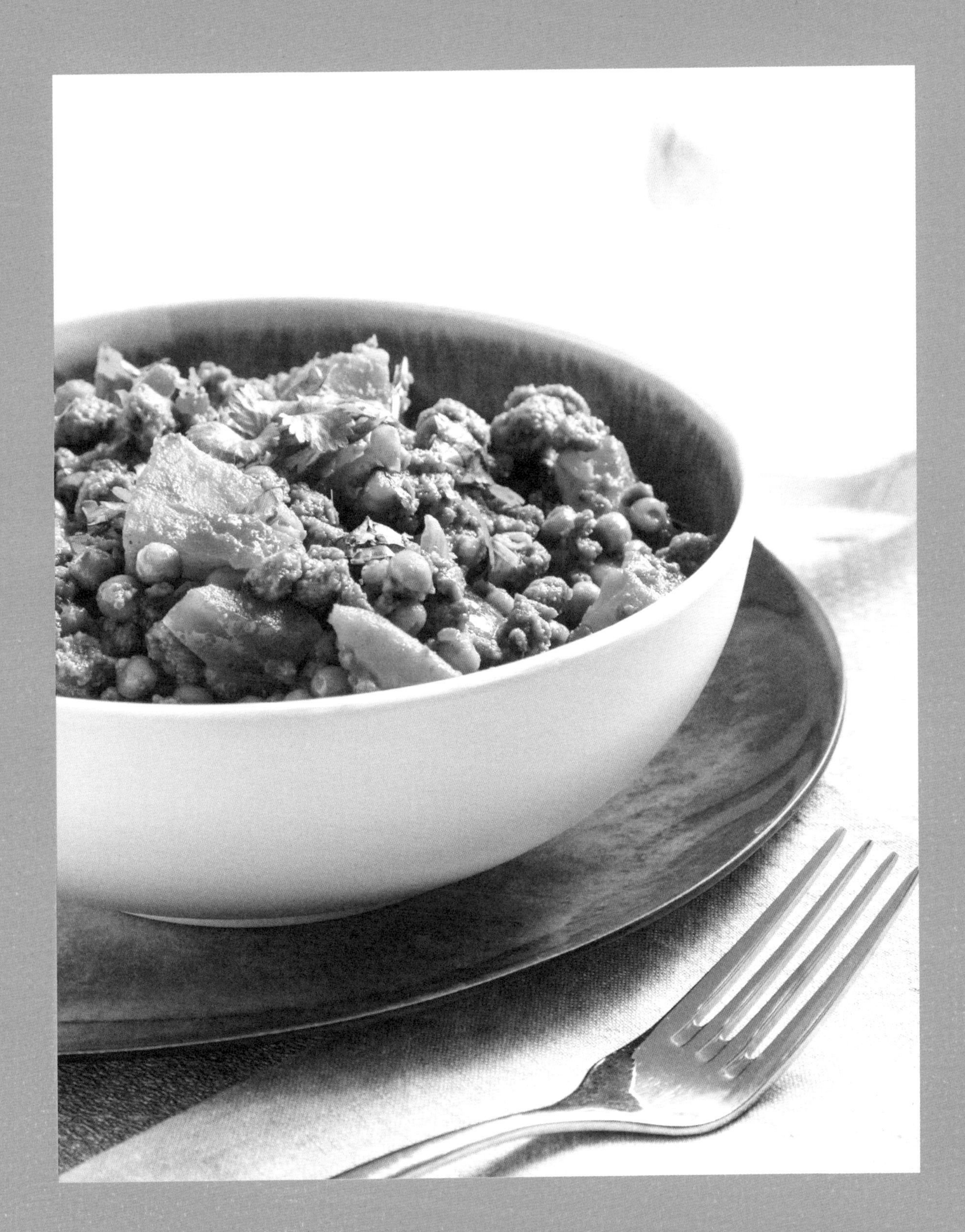

LASAGNE

SERVES TWO

- 2 tsp extra virgin olive oil
- ½ red pepper, deseeded and finely chopped
- 1 large Portobello mushroom, finely chopped
- 2 garlic cloves, crushed
- ½ red onion, finely chopped
- sprinkle of chilli flakes, chilli powder, or fresh chilli (optional)
- 1 tbsp tomato paste
- Quorn mince (grounds), 2 x the size and thickness of your palm
- 12 basil leaves, finely chopped
- pinch of ground white pepper
- 1 tsp Italian mixed herbs
- 1 courgette (zucchini) shaved into wide strips with a potato peeler
- 1 tbsp full-fat cottage cheese
- freshly ground black pepper
- big bunch of rocket leaves (arugala)

This is my healthier take on an Italian classic by replacing the meat element with tasty Quorn and the pasta with courgette. Quorn is a fantastic way to add a plant-based protein to your diet as it contains all the essential amino acids found in animal protein sources.

1. Preheat the oven to 180°C (160°C fan/350°F/Gas 4).
2. In a non-stick frying pan cook the pepper, mushroom, garlic, and red onion in the olive oil on a medium heat for around 3 minutes or until they start to soften (add some chilli here if you want to spice it up).
3. Now add the tomato paste and 100ml (6½ tablespoons) of water and stir well.
4. Add the Quorn mince, basil, white pepper, and Italian mixed herbs, and simmer for around 5 minutes.
5. To assemble, place a layer of shaved courgette strips in a small oven dish and then add half of the Quorn mix. Add another layer of courgette and the rest of the Quorn mix. Top with the remaining courgette strips and, using your fingers, spread the cottage cheese over the top, making sure the courgette is covered.
6. Season with black pepper and bake in the oven for 20 minutes.
7. Divide between two plates and serve with peppery rocket leaves.

CAJUN RAINBOW TROUT

SERVES ONE

- ½ tsp dried thyme
- ½ tsp dried oregano
- ½ tsp ground white pepper
- juice of 1 lime (saving a wedge to garnish)
- 1 rainbow trout fillet, the size and thickness of your palm
- ½ courgette (zucchini), sliced into ribbons
- small handful of mixed leafy salad
- ½ red pepper, deseeded and sliced
- 1 tsp extra virgin olive oil
- freshly ground black pepper

If you are wondering how to add more fish to your diet, then try this recipe, which is simple to follow and absolutely delicious. The sweet, delicate flavour of the rainbow trout is complimented well by the spicy Cajun rub.

1. Place a baking tray in the oven and heat to 180°C (160°C fan/350°F/Gas 4).
2. While the oven is warming, create the spicy Cajun rub by combining the thyme and oregano with the white pepper and half of the lime juice in a bowl and mixing thoroughly.
3. Gently cover the trout with the Cajun rub and bake in the oven for 15 minutes or until cooked through.
4. While the trout is baking, make the salad. Add the courgette, mixed salad leaves, and red pepper to a bowl, and mix with the rest of the lime juice.
5. To serve, add everything to a plate and then drizzle over the olive oil, season with black pepper, and garnish with the wedge of lime.

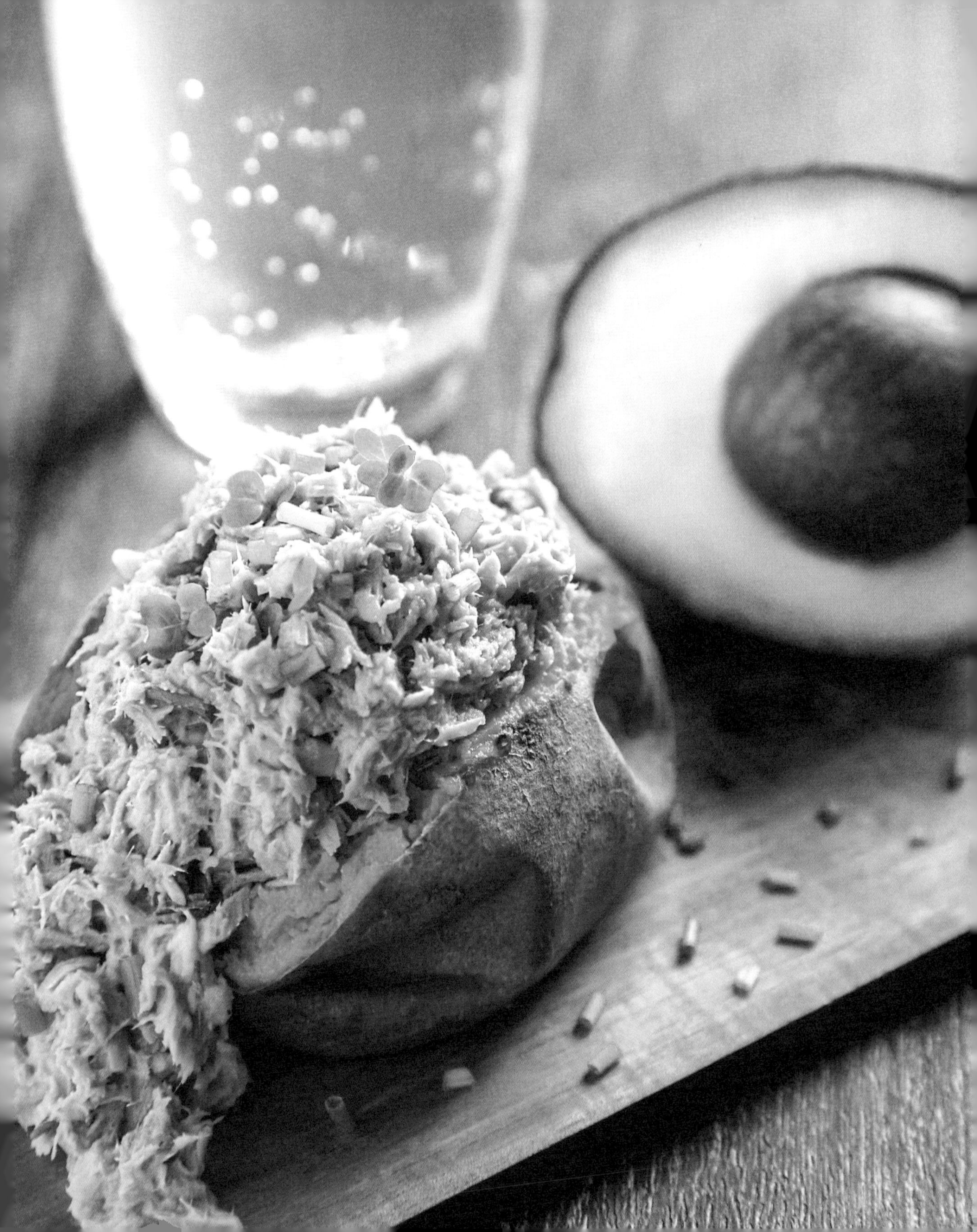

JACKET POTATO WITH TUNA AVONNAISE

SERVES ONE

- 1 small sweet potato
- ½ avocado
- canned tuna in spring water, the size and thickness of your palm, drained
- 1 tsp full-fat Greek yogurt OR Greek-style soya-based vegan yogurt
- juice of ½ lime
- 1 tsp fresh, finely chopped chives, plus a little extra to garnish

We all know consuming fish as part of your diet provides multiple benefits, from improving the condition of your skin and hair to keeping your heart healthy. By regularly adding tuna to your diet you are helping your body maintain a healthy blood pressure, strengthen your immune system and keep your bones strong. Replacing regular mayo with a mix of avocado and Greek yogurt, gives you the creaminess of mayo with heart-healthy unsaturated fats instead of saturated.

1. Preheat the oven to 180°C (160°C fan/350°F/Gas 4).
2. Prick the sweet potato all over with a fork, place it on a baking tray and bake for 40 minutes or until crispy on the outside and soft in the middle.
3. Meanwhile, prepare the tuna topping.
4. In a bowl, mash the avocado, then add the tuna, yogurt, lime juice, and chives. Mix, cover, and put in the fridge until the potato is cooked.
5. When the potato is fluffy on the inside, slice it lengthways and pinch to open. Fill it with the tuna avonnaise and garnish with the chopped chives.

TURKEY MEATBALLS AND STIR-FRY VEGETABLES

SERVES TWO

- lean turkey mince (ground turkey), 2 x the size and thickness of your palm
- 2 garlic cloves, crushed
- ½ small red onion, finely chopped
- handful of fresh, chopped coriander (cilantro), plus a little extra to garnish
- 1 tsp ground coriander
- 1 tsp ground cumin
- pinch of ground white pepper
- ½ tsp paprika
- zest of 1 lemon
- 1 egg, beaten
- 2 tsp extra virgin olive oil
- 1 red pepper, deseeded and chopped
- 1 large courgette (zucchini), sliced
- 1 large red onion, chopped
- squeeze of lemon

Turkey is such a lean, versatile meat, rich in protein and easy to find minced. You could replace it with a vegan mince, if you prefer. I love the way the spices come together in this dish and it proves you don't have to spend hours cooking to make a tasty and healthy meal.

1. Preheat the oven to 180°C (160°C fan/350°F/Gas 4).
2. In a large bowl, mix together the turkey, garlic, red onion, fresh coriander, ground coriander, cumin, white pepper, paprika, lemon, and egg.
3. Shape the mixture into small ball shapes by rolling it between your hands.
4. Place the meatballs on a baking tray and cook in the oven for 15 minutes, turning frequently. They may take slightly longer if you have made larger meatballs.
5. Meanwhile, heat the olive oil in a non-stick frying pan or wok and stir-fry the pepper, courgette, and onion until they are cooked to your liking.
6. To serve, place the vegetables in bowls and add the cooked meatballs on top. Garnish with some fresh coriander and a squeeze of lemon juice.

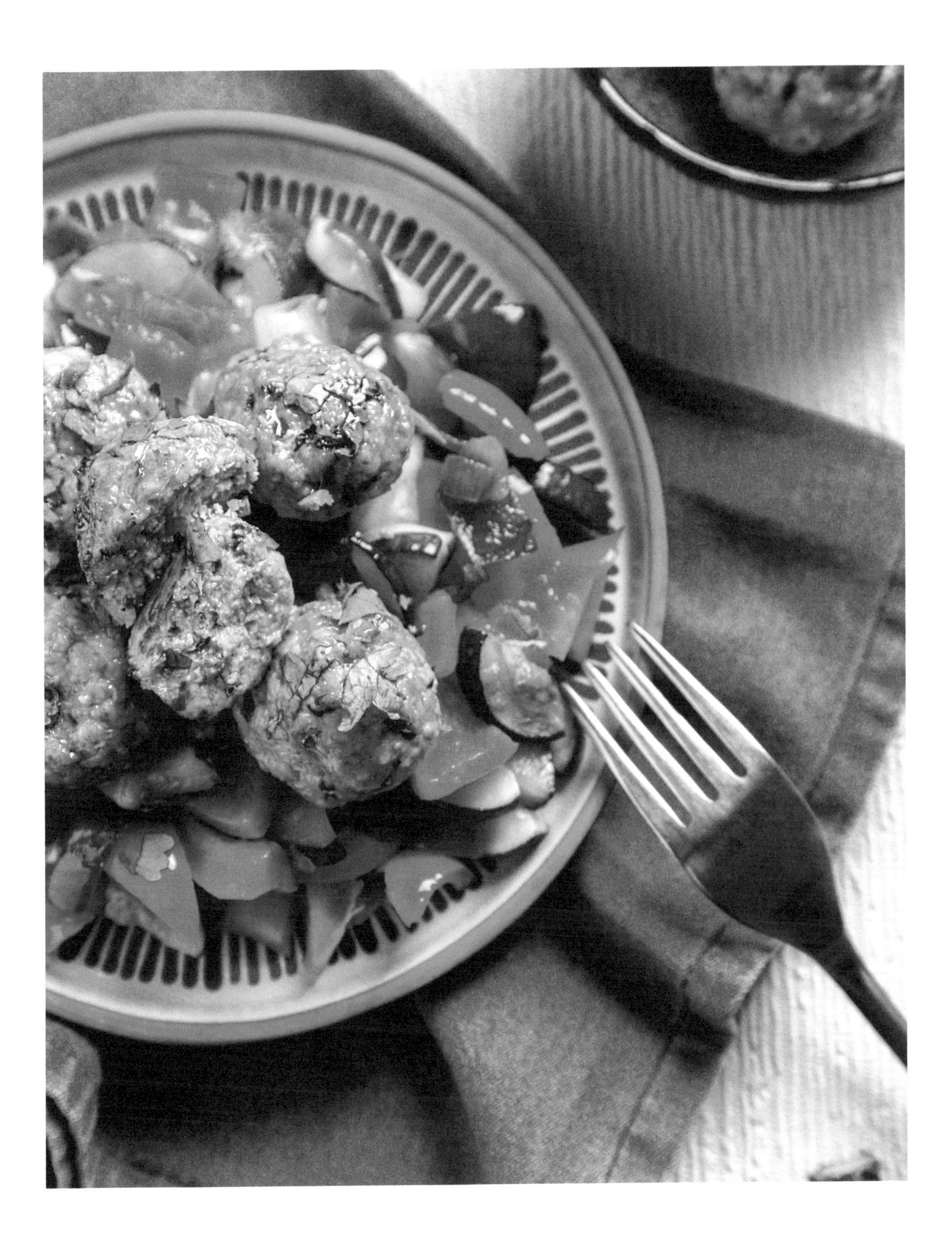

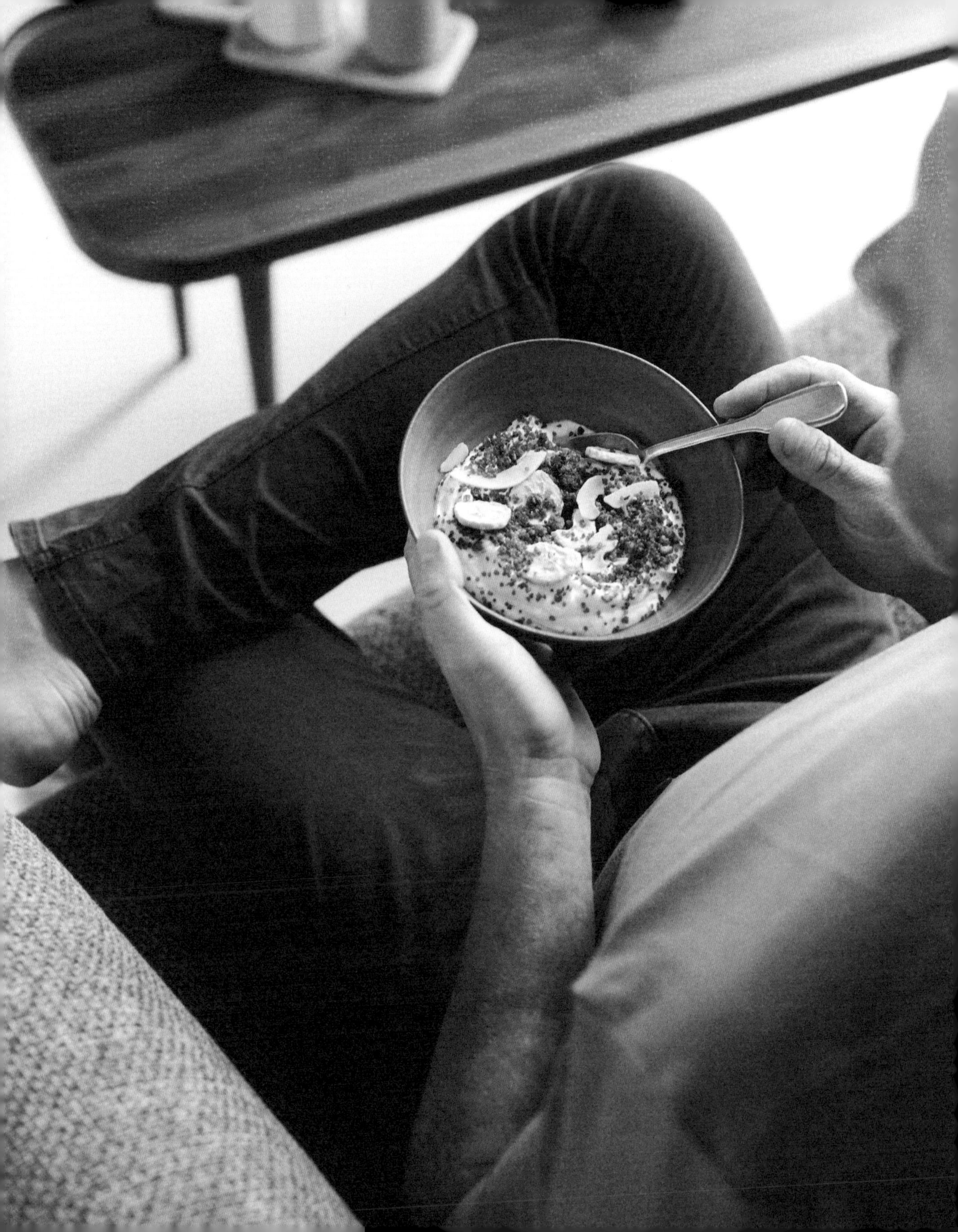

SNACKS

Welcome to my collection of healthy snacks, where delicious meets nutritious. Enjoy these wholesome snacks that not only satisfy your cravings but also fuel your body with goodness.

CHERRY AND VANILLA SHAKE

SERVES ONE

- handful of pitted frozen cherries
- 3 tbsp full-fat Greek yogurt OR Greek-style soya (soy)-based vegan yogurt
- 200ml (scant 1 cup) unsweetened soya (soy) milk OR unsweetened pea milk
- 2 tsp chia seeds
- 1 vanilla pod

You don't need to wait until cherries come into their short season, you can enjoy this super easy shake all year round by using frozen cherries. You may have noticed that many of my recipes, especially my shakes and smoothies, contain chia seeds. These tiny little super seeds are now readily available in most supermarkets and can be stored in the cupboard and added to any meal to provide an abundance of nutrients to your daily diet.

1. Put the cherries, yogurt, and soya or pea milk in a blender and blitz until smooth.
2. Add the chia seeds and the vanilla pod seeds (scrape these out of the middle of the pod by scoring then scraping with a knife), then blitz again until completely smooth.
3. To cool the shake, add some ice and blitz until crushed.
4. Poor into a tall glass, top with a cherry, and enjoy or have as an on-the-go breakfast or snack.

GOOD TO KNOW

Since most frozen fruits are frozen shortly after they are harvested, they're allowed to fully ripen, which means they're packed full of vitamins and antioxidants as freezing them "locks all the goodness in". Drop the empty vanilla pod in some boiled water to make vanilla tea.

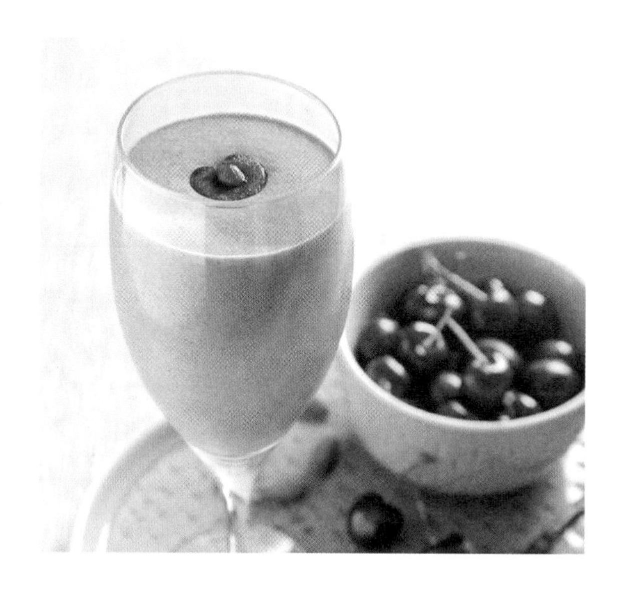

BLACKBERRY AND COCONUT SMOOTHIE

SERVES ONE

200ml (scant 1 cup) unsweetened soya (soy) milk or unsweetened pea milk

3 tbsp full-fat Greek yogurt OR Greek-style soya (soy)-based vegan yogurt

handful of frozen mixed berries

2 tsp desiccated (flaked) coconut

This is an old favourite of mine; you can see at a glance that it's extraordinarily simple, but the full-on flavour of the coconut combined with the fruit has a gratifying complexity. The addition of coconut adds essential nutrients and healthy fats to your diet.

1 Add the unsweetened soya or pea milk, the yogurt, and the berries to a blender and blitz until smooth.

2 Add the coconut, a handful of ice and blitz again.

3 Pour into a tall glass or your "on the go" drinks bottle and enjoy this smoothie as your breakfast or as a snack.

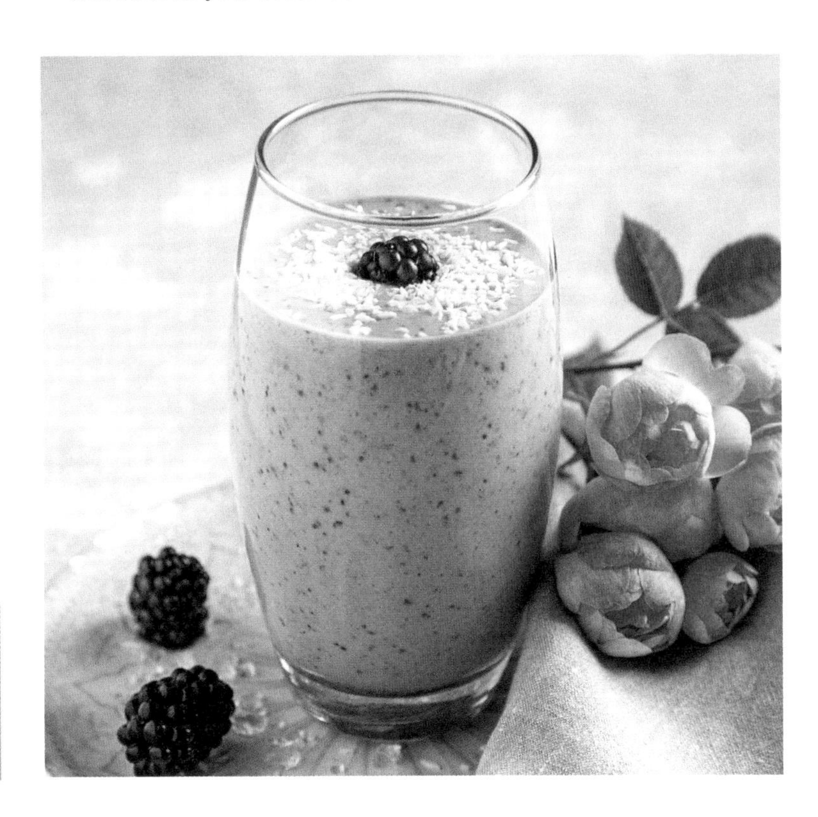

GOOD TO KNOW

Use frozen mixed fruit from the supermarket, it's still packed full of nutrients and is often cheaper.

KEY LIME PIE SMOOTHIE

SERVES ONE

- 1 rice cake
- 1 tbsp oats
- ½ serving of The Six Pack Revolution Vanilla Caramel Heaven Post Workout Protein Shake Powder
- 150ml (⅔ cup) unsweetened almond milk
- juice and zest of 1 lime (reserve a thin slice to decorate)
- 6 cashew nuts, chopped or finely crushed

Tart, sharp, and sweet! My key lime pie smoothie is made from just a handful of delicious ingredients, perfect for an "anytime of the day" treat!

1 Crush the rice cake and put to one side.

2 Add all remaining ingredients and a handful of ice to a blender and blitz until smooth.

3 Sprinkle the crushed rice cake on the top of the smoothie and decorate with a slice of lime, if you wish.

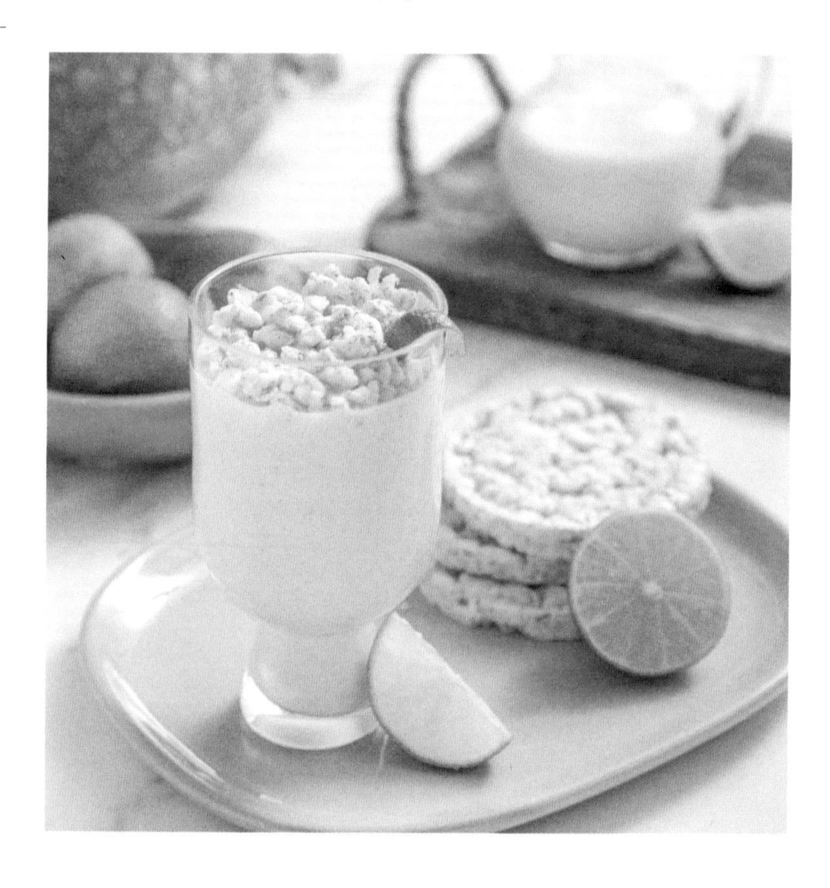

RASPBERRY RIPPLE SMOOTHIE

SERVES ONE

- 1 tbsp full-fat cottage cheese
- 2 tbsp full-fat Greek yogurt OR Greek-style soya (soy)-based vegan yogurt
- 200ml (scant 1 cup) unsweetened soya (soy) milk OR unsweetened pea milk
- zest of ½ lemon
- squeeze of lemon juice
- seeds of 1 vanilla pod
- handful of raspberries (fresh or frozen)

My daughter absolutely loves this healthy smoothie and it is super cute when served in little milk bottle-style glass jars with a straw. Seriously though, this smoothie is perfect for everyone and tastes delicious.

1. Add all the ingredients and a handful of ice to a blender and blitz.
2. Serve in your favourite glass or shaker and enjoy.

GOOD TO KNOW

Add the empty pod in some boiling water for a vanilla twist to your tea.

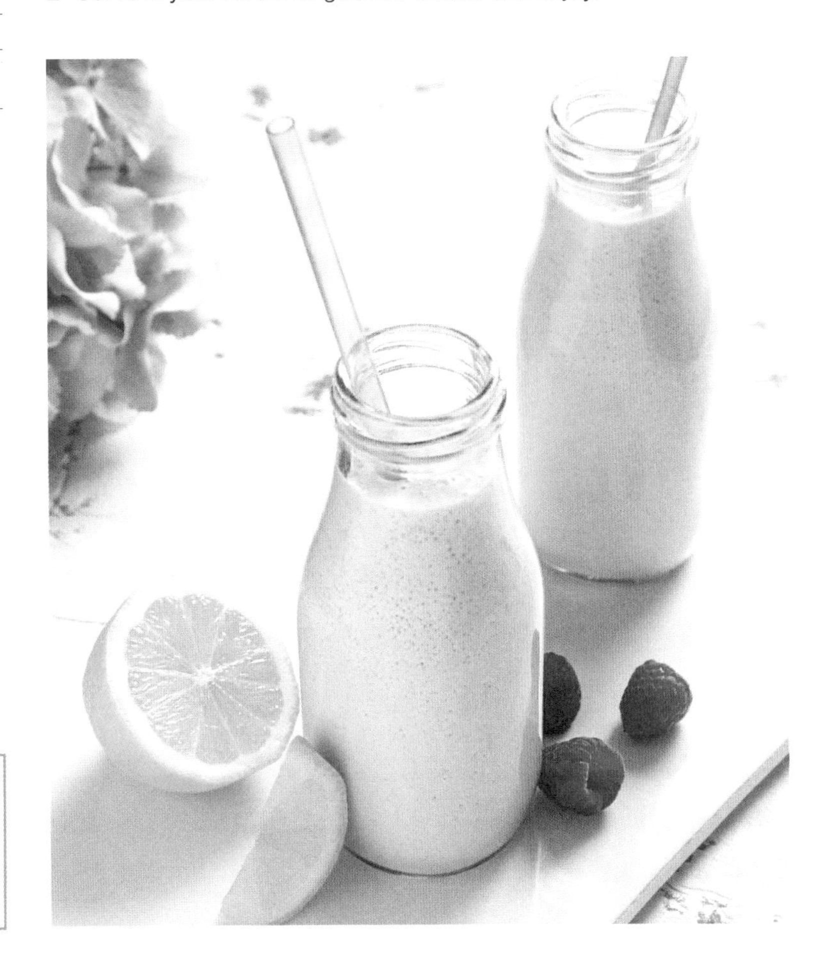

MINT CHOCOLATE MILKSHAKE

SERVES ONE

- ½ banana
- small handful of fresh spinach
- small handful of fresh blueberries
- 1 tbsp fresh mint leaves, plus a sprig to decorate
- 300ml (1¼ cup) unsweetened soya (soy) milk OR unsweetened pea milk
- 1½ tbsp organic cacao powder

Chocolate and mint; the perfect flavour combination – not just for after dinner as this is a snack you can enjoy any time of the day. The added spinach and blueberries, or brain berries as I like to call them, means this milkshake has some serious health benefits.

1. Add all the ingredients and a handful of ice to a blender and blitz into a smooth consistency.
2. Pour into your favourite glass and decorate with a sprig of mint.

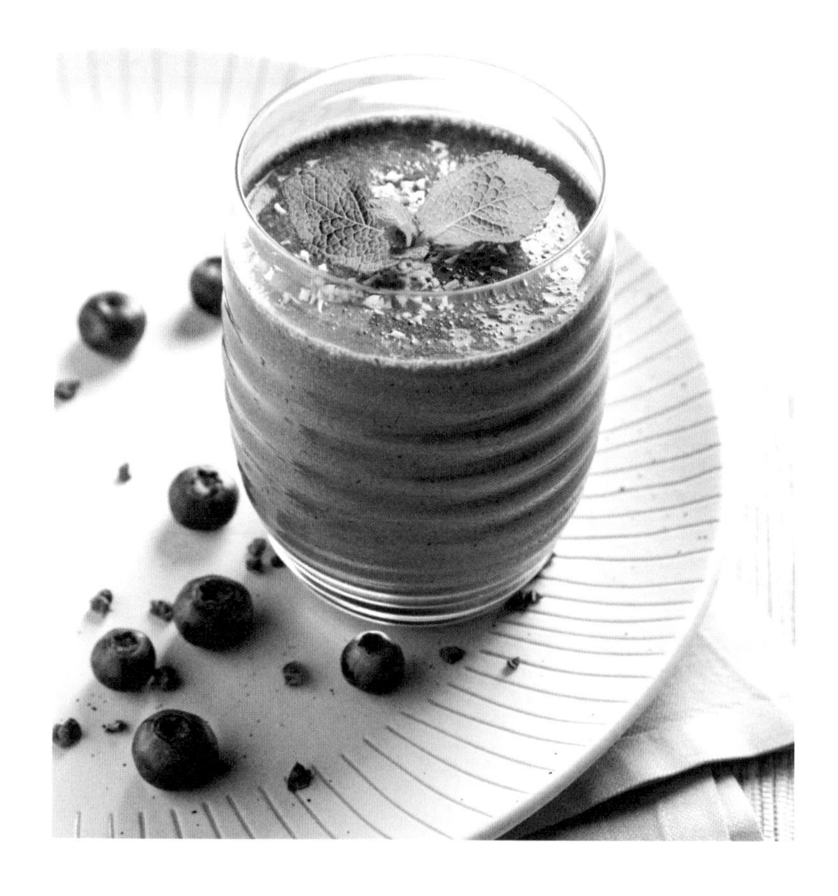

SWEET POTATO AND BANANA PANCAKES

SERVES ONE

- handful of sweet potato, peeled and cut into cubes
- 1 banana
- 3 eggs
- splash of unsweetened soya (soy) milk or unsweetened pea milk
- pinch of cinnamon
- 1 tsp coconut oil
- juice of ½ a lemon (optional)
- 1 tbsp full-fat Greek yogurt OR Greek-style soya (soy)-based vegan yogurt

These truly are my tastiest, fluffiest pancakes, and the kids love them too. On top of that, they are super healthy and a surprisingly sweet delight.

1. Bring a pot of water to the boil and cook the sweet potato for 15 minutes or until they are soft. Drain and mash the potato together with half the banana.
2. In a blender, beat the eggs for 1 minute, then add the mash, the soya or pea milk, and the cinnamon.
3. Now heat the coconut oil in a frying pan and add the batter to make one pancake at a time. Cook for a few minutes on each side, then remove from the pan.
4. Transfer the pancakes to a plate, add a squeeze of lemon if you like, then finely slice the remaining banana and serve on top of the pancake with the yogurt.

VEGAN STRAWBERRY PANCAKES

SERVES ONE

- 4 tbsp gram (chickpea) flour
- 1 scoop of The Six Pack Revolution Vegan Strawberry Cream Sensation Post Workout Protein Shake Powder
- ½ tsp baking powder
- 1 tsp coconut oil
- 1 tbsp Greek-style soya (soy)-based vegan yogurt
- small handful of strawberries, sliced

Fluffy, strawberrylicious pancakes, perfect for snacking all day, every day! Never miss a pancake day again with these healthy dollops of goodness. Batch cook and freeze in advance for an always-available anytime snack.

1. Thoroughly mix the dry ingredients together in a bowl. Gradually add 200ml (scant 1 cup) of water, folding the mixture with a spoon to make a wet batter, then set it aside for 5 minutes.
2. Heat a little of the coconut oil in a non-stick frying pan, then add some of the batter to the pan (the size of the pancakes is your choice, they can be as large as the pan or the size of your palm). Leave the batter to cook for a few minutes until the edges are firm, then turn the pancake over and cook the other side until they brown.
3. Continue making pancakes until the batter is used up. Serve the pancakes on a plate with the yogurt and strawberries.

GOOD TO KNOW

A good non-stick pan is very important as you are using a small amount of oil.

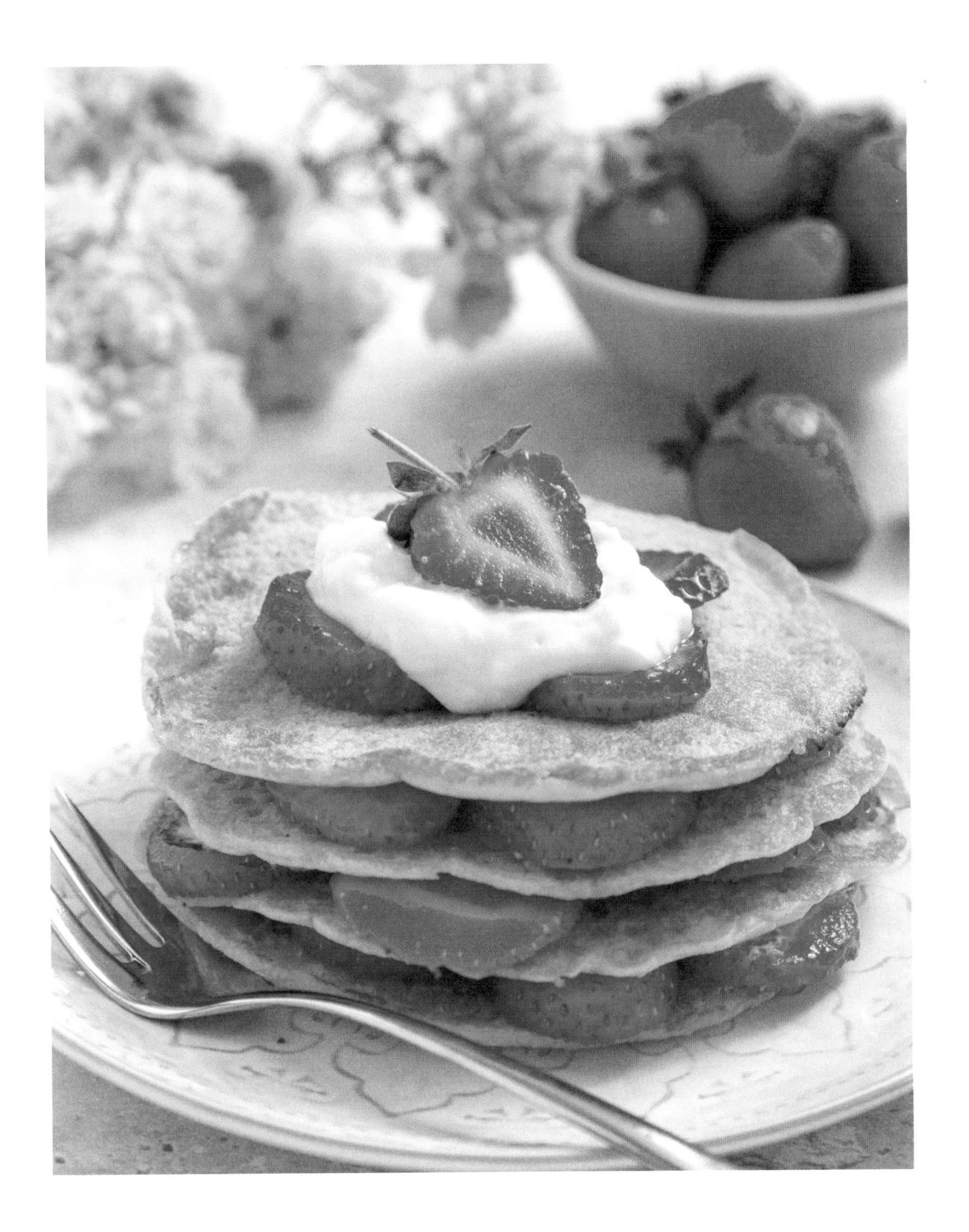

PINEAPPLE PANCAKES WITH COCONUT

SERVES ONE

4 egg whites

1 vanilla pod

2 tbsp oats, blitzed into a powder

handful of fresh pineapple, chopped

3 tbsp full-fat cottage cheese

1 tsp coconut oil

TO SERVE

1 tsp full-fat Greek yogurt OR Greek-style soya (soy)-based vegan yogurt

1 tbsp coconut flakes OR desiccated coconut

By adding the tropical flavours of pineapple and coconut, you are taking the humble pancake to the next level of deliciousness. These are best served warm, letting the juices of the fresh pineapple soak into the pancakes.

1. Remove the seeds from the vanilla pod (scrape these out of the middle of the pod by scoring then scraping with a knife).
2. Add the egg whites and vanilla pod seeds to a blender and whizz until frothy.
3. Add the oats and half the pineapple, blend again, then fold in the cottage cheese.
4. Heat a non-stick frying pan and add a little of the coconut oil.
5. Pour a quarter of the pancake mixture into the pan, leave it to set for a few minutes, then flip it over and cook the other side. Transfer to a plate and keep it warm under a low grill (broiler). Repeat for the other three pancakes.
6. Pile the pancakes on a plate and serve topped with the rest of the fresh pineapple, the yogurt and coconut.

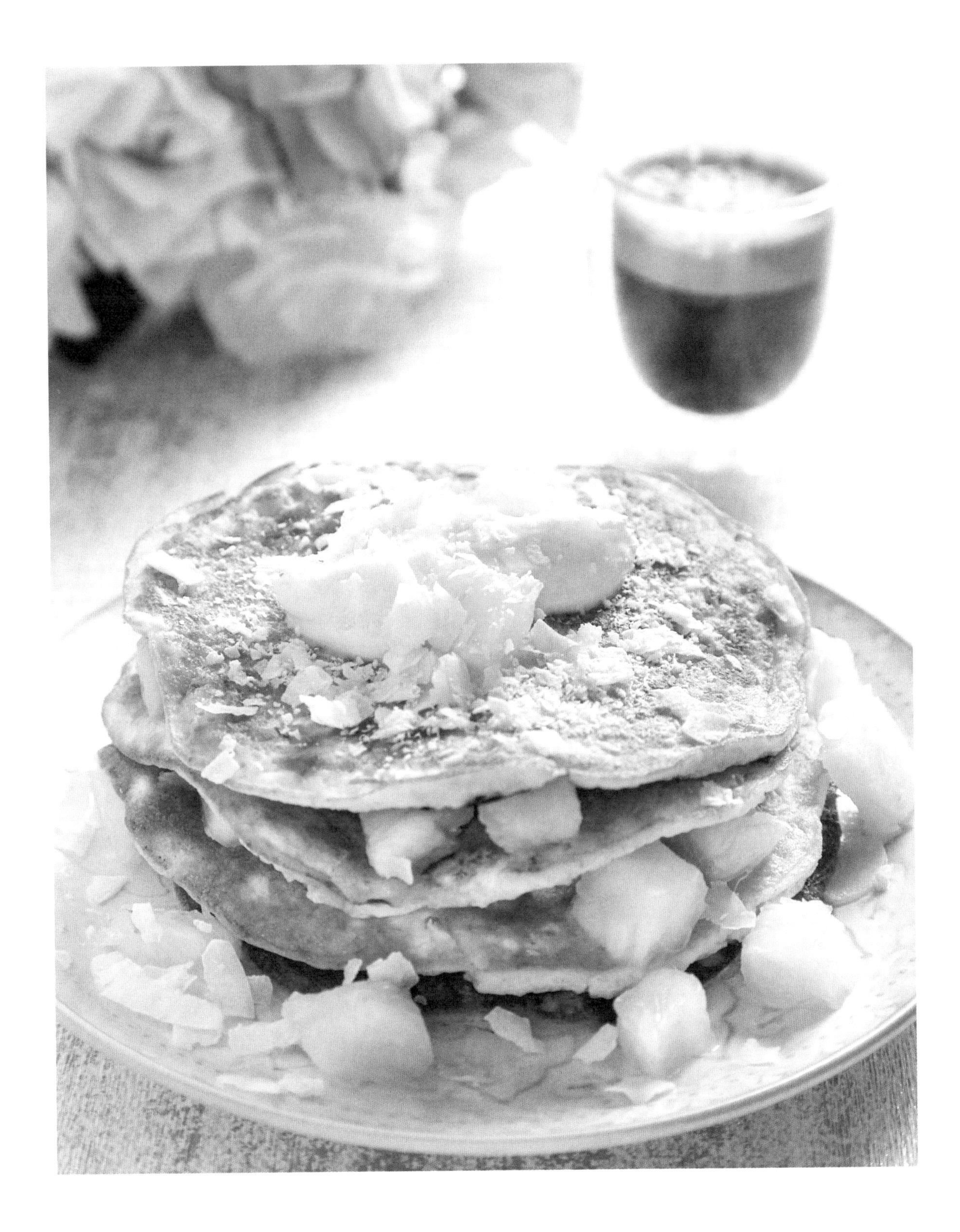

DOUBLE CHOCOLATE AND HAZELNUT QUINOLA

SERVES TWO

- 250g (9oz) cooked or 80g (3oz) dry quinoa
- 1 tbsp chia seeds
- 1 tbsp cacao nibs
- 12 hazelnuts, roughly chopped
- ½ serving of The Six Pack Revolution Decadent Chocolate Caramel Post Workout Protein Shake Powder
- 1 tsp honey

TO SERVE

- 3 tbsp full-fat Greek yogurt OR Greek-style soya (soy)-based vegan yogurt OR 200ml (scant 1 cup) unsweetened soya (soy) milk OR unsweetened pea milk

Snack any time of the day on this little beaut! Not only delicious and healthy, you can keep the quinola mixture in an airtight container to enjoy again and again. Bonus!

1. Preheat the oven to 140°C (120°C fan/275°F/Gas 1).
2. Cook the quinoa, following the packet instructions, drain, then set aside to cool.
3. To make the quinola mixture, add the cooked quinoa, chia seeds, cacao nibs, hazelnuts, and protein powder to a bowl then mix together well.
4. Add the honey and mix everything together with your hands, making sure the honey coats all the mixture.
5. Transfer the mixture to a baking tray lined with baking parchment and spread out evenly.
6. Place the tray in the middle of the oven and cook for 30 minutes, checking every 10 minutes, stirring and folding each time. The mixture should be browned all over but take care not to burn it.
7. Take it out of the oven and leave to cool. Eat straight away or store in an airtight container for up to 2 weeks. Serve with 3 tablespoons of yogurt, soya, or pea milk per portion.

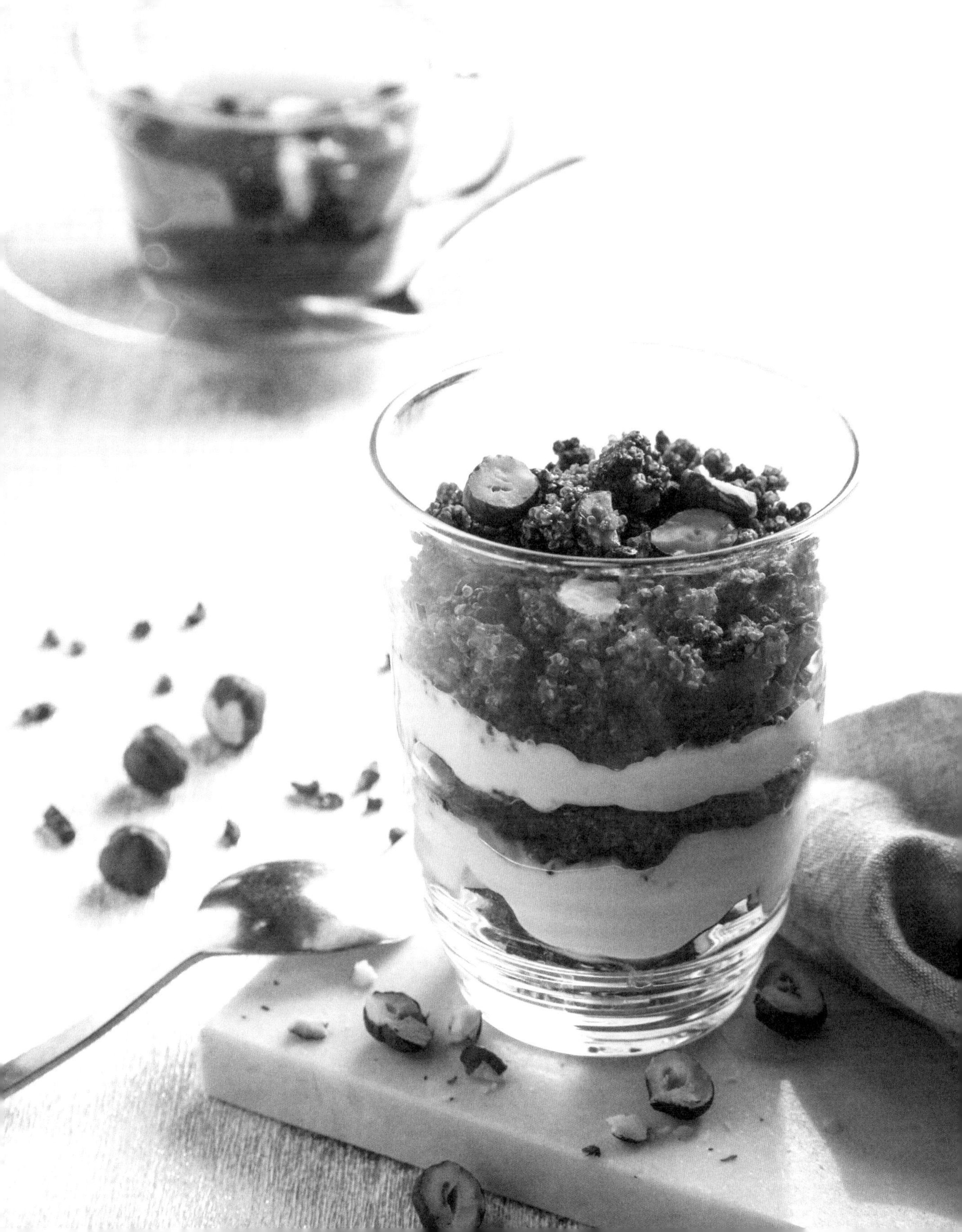

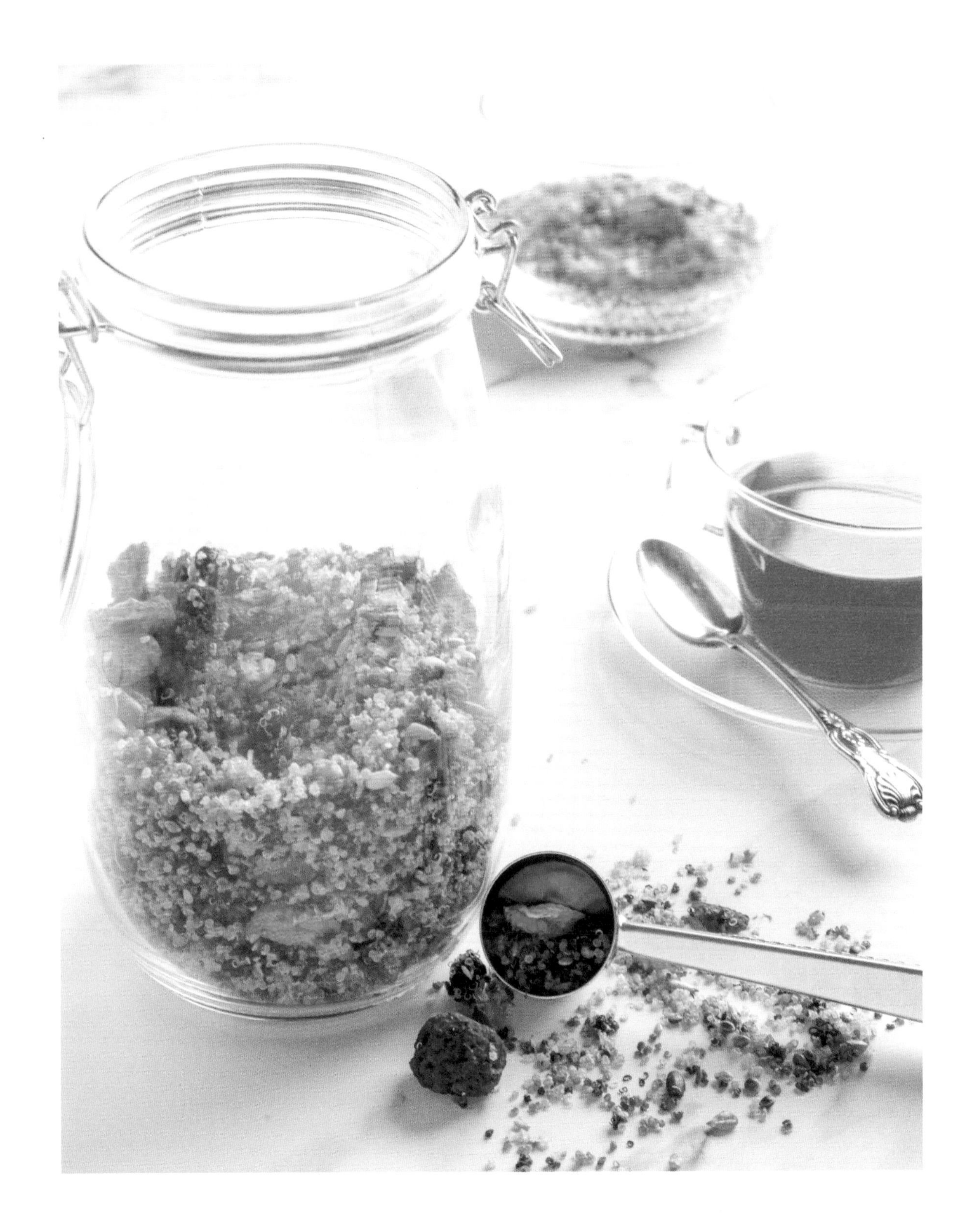

MIXED BERRY QUINOLA

SERVES TWO

250g (9oz) cooked or 80g (3oz) dry quinoa

1 tbsp chia seeds

1 tbsp mixed seeds (such as sunflower seeds, flaxseeds, and poppy seeds)

12 pecan halves, crushed

1 generous tsp honey

1 heaped tbsp freeze-dried blueberries

1 heaped tbsp freeze-dried raspberries

TO SERVE

3 tbsp full-fat Greek yogurt OR Greek-style soya (soy)-based vegan yogurt OR 200ml (scant 1 cup) unsweetened soya (soy) milk OR unsweetened pea milk

This sticky, nutty, crunchy super-healthy quinola literally bursts with flavour from the addition of freeze-dried fruit.

1. Preheat the oven to 140°C (120°C fan/275°F/Gas 1).
2. To make the quinola, add the cooked quinoa, seeds, and pecans to a bowl and stir together.
3. Add the honey and mix everything together with your hands, making sure the honey coats the mixture.
4. Transfer the mixture to a baking tray lined with baking parchment and spread out evenly.
5. Place the tray in the middle of the oven and cook for 30 minutes, checking every 10 minutes, stirring and folding each time. When it's browned but not burnt, remove the baking tray from the oven and leave to cool completely. You can leave it in the switched-off oven overnight for it to go extra crunchy. Add the freeze-dried fruit to the mixture, making sure it's mixed well.
6. Eat straight away or store in an airtight container for up to 2 weeks. Serve with 3 tablespoons of yogurt, soya, or pea milk per portion.

BANANA AND COCONUT QUINOLA

SERVES TWO

250g (9oz) cooked or 80g (3oz) dry quinoa

2 tsp mixed seeds (such as sunflower seeds, flaxseeds, and poppy seeds)

2 heaped tbsp freeze-dried banana

2 tsp coconut flakes

1 tsp honey

TO SERVE

3 tbsp full-fat Greek yogurt OR Greek-style soya (soy)-based vegan yogurt OR 200ml (scant 1 cup) unsweetened soya (soy) OR pea milk

Anytime is the ideal time for this! Full of potassium and fibre – courtesy of the banana, and healthy fats from the coconut… this snack is great from morning to night.

1. Preheat the oven to 140°C (120°C fan/275°F/Gas 1).
2. Add the cooked quinoa and mixed seeds to a bowl and stir together.
3. Add the honey and mix everything together with your hands, making sure the honey coats the mixture.
4. Transfer the mixture to a baking tray lined with greaseproof paper and spread it out evenly.
5. Place the baking tray in the middle of the oven for 30 minutes. Check it every 10 minutes, stirring, and folding it all together each time. When it's browned but not burnt remove the baking tray from the oven and leave to cool completely. You can leave it in the switched-off oven overnight for it to go extra crunchy.
6. Finally, add the freeze-dried banana and coconut flakes to the cooled mixture.
7. Eat straight away or store in an airtight container for up to 2 weeks. Serve with 3 tablespoons of yogurt, soya, or pea milk per portion.

COTTAGE CHEESE WITH BLUEBERRY AND COCONUT

SERVES ONE

3 tbsp full-fat cottage cheese
handful of blueberries
2 tsp desiccated (flaked) coconut

I love this quick and easy recipe. Blueberries are low in calories but high in nutrients and while the cottage cheese in this dish may seem a strange addition, surprisingly it's a combination that works. The flavour of the coconut makes this wonderfully simple recipe come alive, so give it a go and try something a little different.

1 Add everything to a bowl and serve.

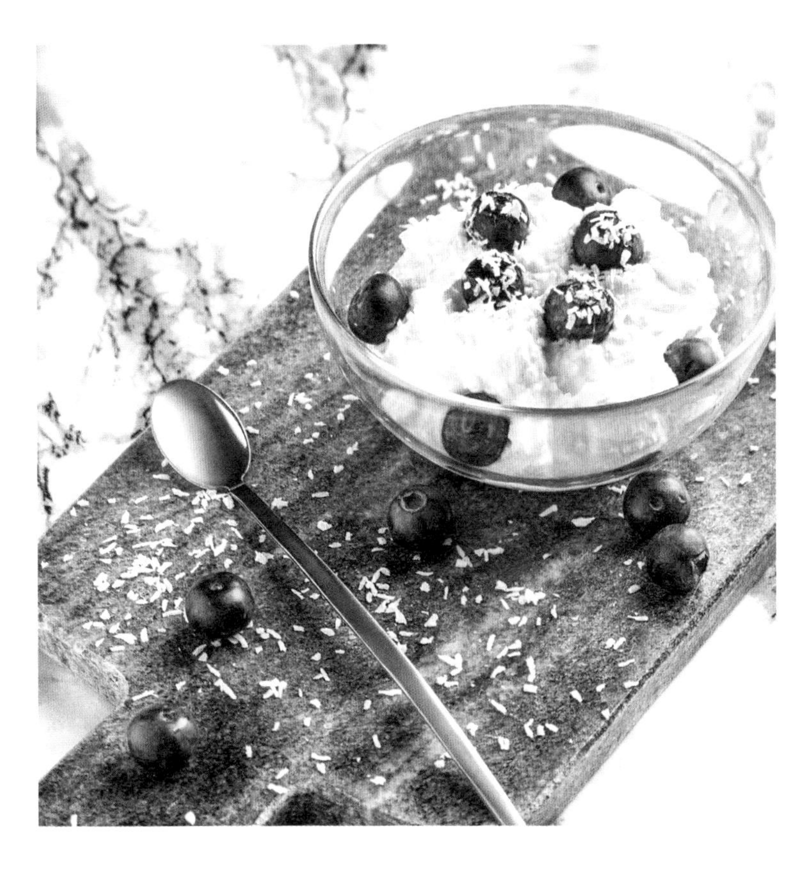

PLANT-BASED PORRIDGE WITH BLUEBERRIES

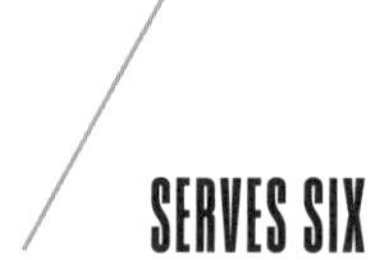

SERVES SIX

90g (scant ¾ cup) oats
4 tbsp barley flakes
3 tbsp uncooked quinoa
2 tbsp chia seeds
1 tbsp dried cranberries
1 tbsp dried blueberries
36 unsalted almonds, chopped (reserve a few for decoration)
1 tsp cinnamon

FOR EACH SERVING

200ml (scant 1 cup) unsweetened soya milk OR unsweetened pea milk
6 fresh blueberries

This porridge is easy to make and the uncooked mixture will keep in an airtight container for months, although it's so delicious, I'd be surprised if it lasts that long! The combination of grains adds to the texture, giving it an almost muesli feel.

1. Combine the oats, barley flakes, quinoa, chia seeds, cranberries, blueberries, almonds, and cinnamon thoroughly and store in an airtight container.
2. For each serving, add 3 heaped tablespoons of the porridge mix to a small pan with the soya or pea milk.
3. Bring to the boil, then reduce the heat and simmer for 2 minutes or until the porridge has reached the consistency you like. Transfer to a bowl.
4. Squash the fresh blueberries into a pulp with a fork and spoon it over the porridge with a few chopped almonds to finish.

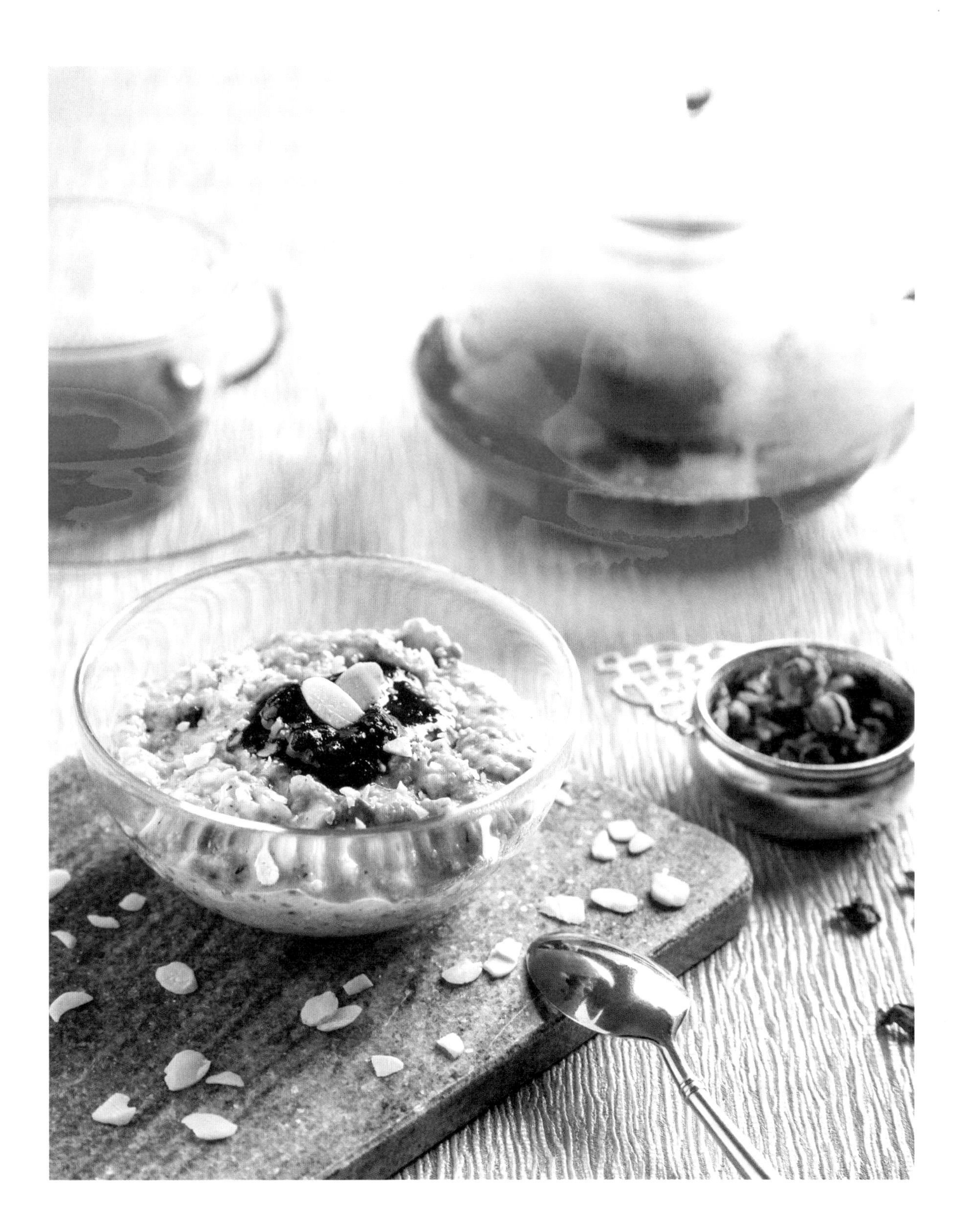

SPANISH OMELETTE WITH PEAS AND ONION

SERVES TWO

- 2 tsp extra virgin olive oil
- handful of sweet potato, peeled and finely sliced
- 1 medium white OR red onion, thinly sliced
- pinch of chilli flakes
- 1 tsp paprika
- handful of frozen peas
- heaped teaspoon of chopped chives
- 4–6 eggs, lightly beaten
- freshly ground black pepper

Treat yourself to a taste of Spain with my easy peasy snack infused with the warmth of chilli flakes and paprika. Bravo!

1. Heat the olive oil in a non-stick frying pan over a low heat. Add the sweet potatoes, put a lid on top and cook for 7–8 minutes, turning often to ensure they do not burn.
2. Now add the onion, chilli flakes, and paprika. Mix everything together carefully and cook for another 3 minutes with the lid on.
3. Add the peas, half the chives, and then the eggs.
4. Season with black pepper and sprinkle the remaining chives over the top.
5. Continue to cook on a low heat for 5 minutes and finish under the grill (broiler) to brown the top, if necessary. Serve immediately or eat cold later.

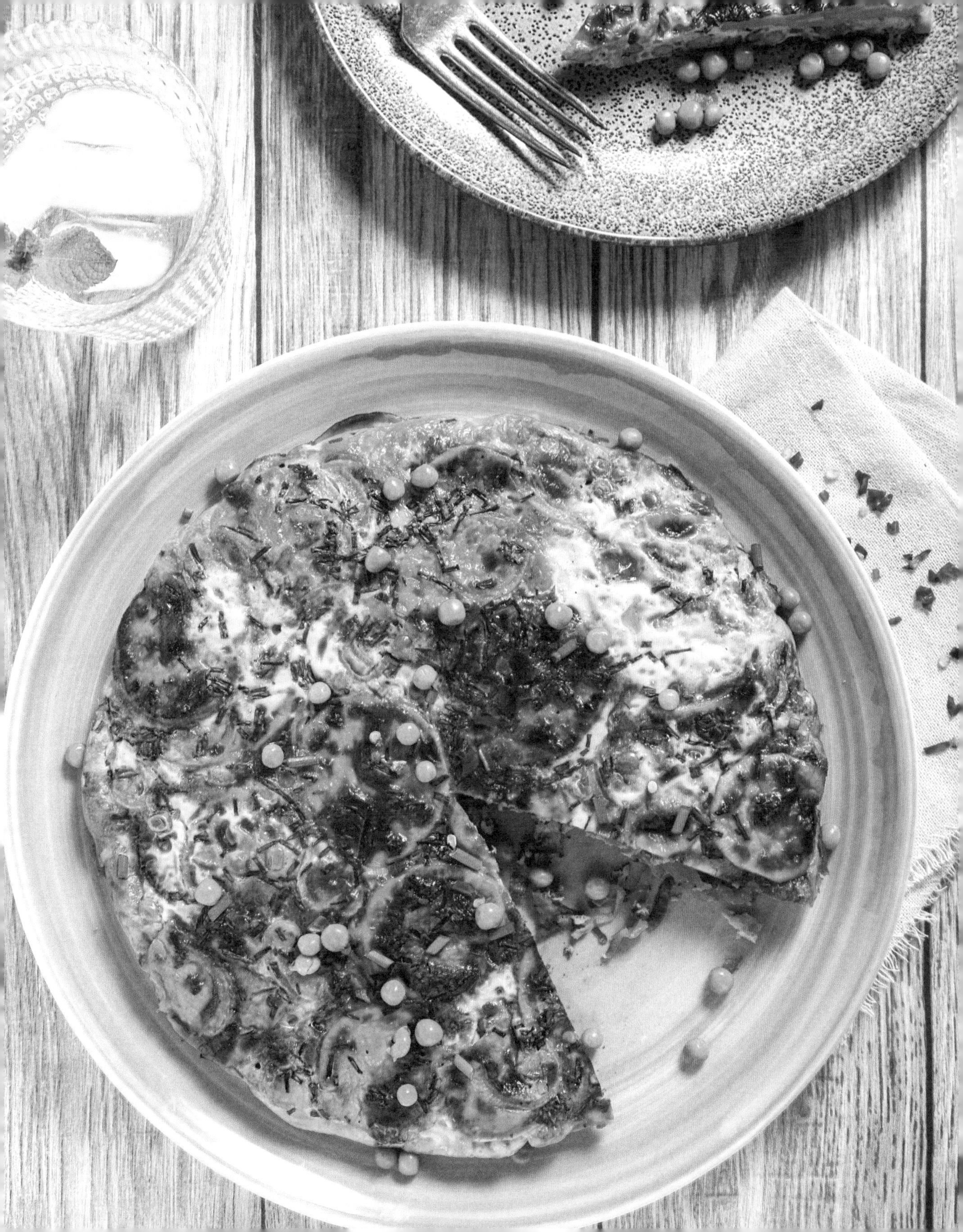

SMOKED MACKEREL PATÉ

SERVES TWO

- 2 smoked mackerel fillets (skin removed)
- ½ avocado
- small handful of fresh coriander (cilantro)
- juice and zest of 1 lime
- ½ tsp mild curry powder
- ½ small apple, grated (skin on)
- 1 wholemeal wrap
- some fresh red chilli, chopped to garnish (optional)

The paté is served with a wholemeal wrap that is divided between two. If you prefer, you can replace the wrap with a couple of sliced carrots (per portion).

1. Add all the ingredients, apart from the wrap and the apple, to a blender and blitz into a smooth paste.
2. Transfer the blitzed ingredients to a bowl, then fold in the grated apple until mixed thoroughly.
3. Dry-fry the wholemeal wrap and cut into triangles. Garnish with coriander and red chilli, if you wish. Dip into the paté and enjoy.

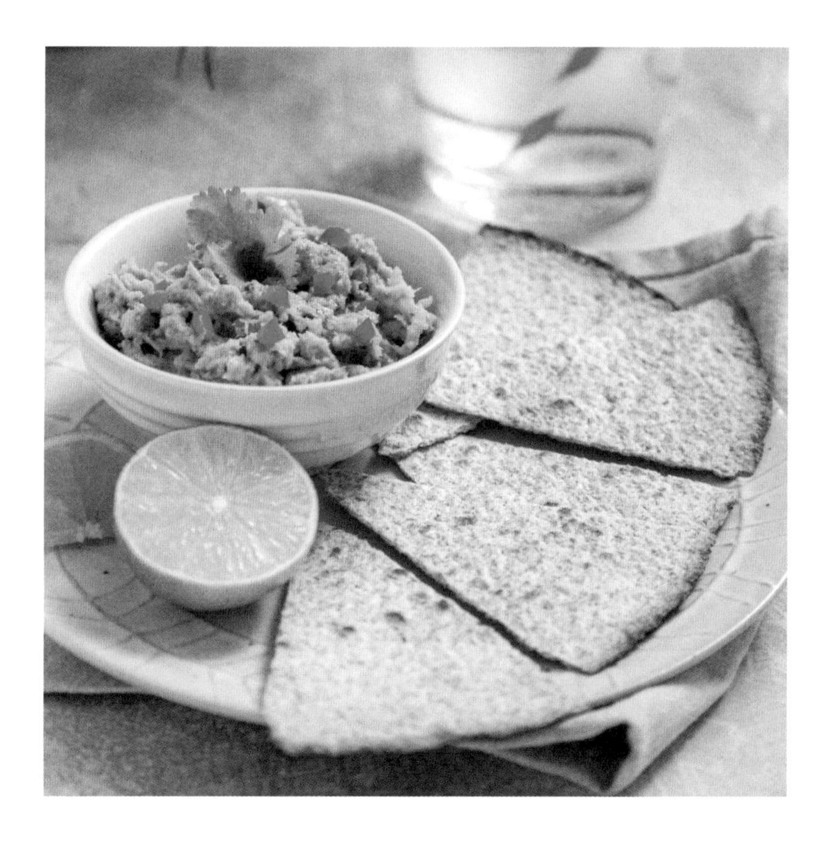

TOMATO AND BASIL OMELETTE

SERVES ONE

- 1 tsp extra virgin olive oil
- 2–3 eggs, lightly beaten
- freshly ground black pepper
- 6 cherry tomatoes, halved
- 8 fresh basil leaves (or to taste)

Together tomato and basil create a classic flavour combination that is simple, fresh, and delicious, making them the perfect filling for an omelette. The aromatic depth of basil complements the superfood, egg, beautifully.

1. Heat the oil gently in a non-stick frying pan, add the beaten eggs, and season with black pepper. Let the egg cook for 2-3 minutes, then turn it over to cook the other side.

2. When the egg is cooked, transfer the omelette to a plate, layer half of it with the tomatoes and basil, then fold the other half over and add a little more black pepper.

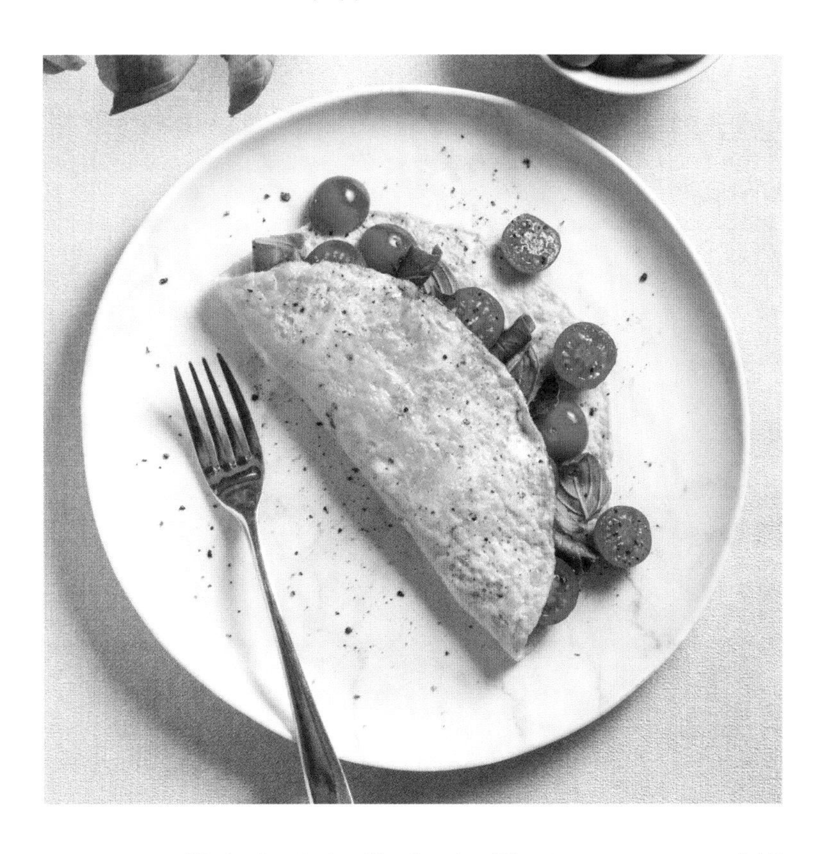

PEA PANCAKES WITH A SPICY MINT SAUCE

SERVES ONE

- 2 tbsp frozen peas
- 4 egg whites
- 3 tbsp oats, blitzed into a powder
- small handful of fresh spinach
- 1 tsp extra virgin olive oil
- 2 tbsp spicy mint sauce
- fresh green chilli, sliced (optional)

FOR THE SPICY MINT SAUCE

- handful of fresh, finely chopped coriander (cilantro)
- handful fresh, finely chopped mint
- juice and zest of ½ lemon
- ½ tsp cumin seeds
- 1 fresh green chilli, deseeded and finely chopped
- 1 garlic clove, crushed
- 2 spring (green) onions, chopped
- 3 tbsp full-fat Greek yogurt OR Greek-style soya (soy)-based vegan yogurt

Peas are healthy, versatile, and taste great, plus they are low in sugars and high in fibre. I like these pancakes as they are perfect for the whole family and really quick to make.

1. Remove the peas from the freezer and allow them to slightly defrost by adding them to a cup and covering with water.
2. To make the spicy mint sauce, put all the ingredients into a blender and blitz. Set aside for the moment.
3. In a blender, blitz the egg whites until they start to fluff up, then add the oats and spinach and blitz again until mixed through. Pour the mixture into a bowl.
4. Drain the peas, add them to the bowl along with the olive oil, and fold them into the mixture.
5. Heat a non-stick frying pan on a medium heat and pour 3–4 small pancake-size amounts of the batter into the centre of the pan. As the batter is quite thick you should be able to shape them with a spoon.
6. Serve the pancakes with spicy mint sauce. Top with a few slices of fresh chilli (if using).

GOOD TO KNOW

Put in an airtight container and it will last in the fridge for a few days or, alternatively, you can freeze it in a couple of separate freezer bags and it will last a month.

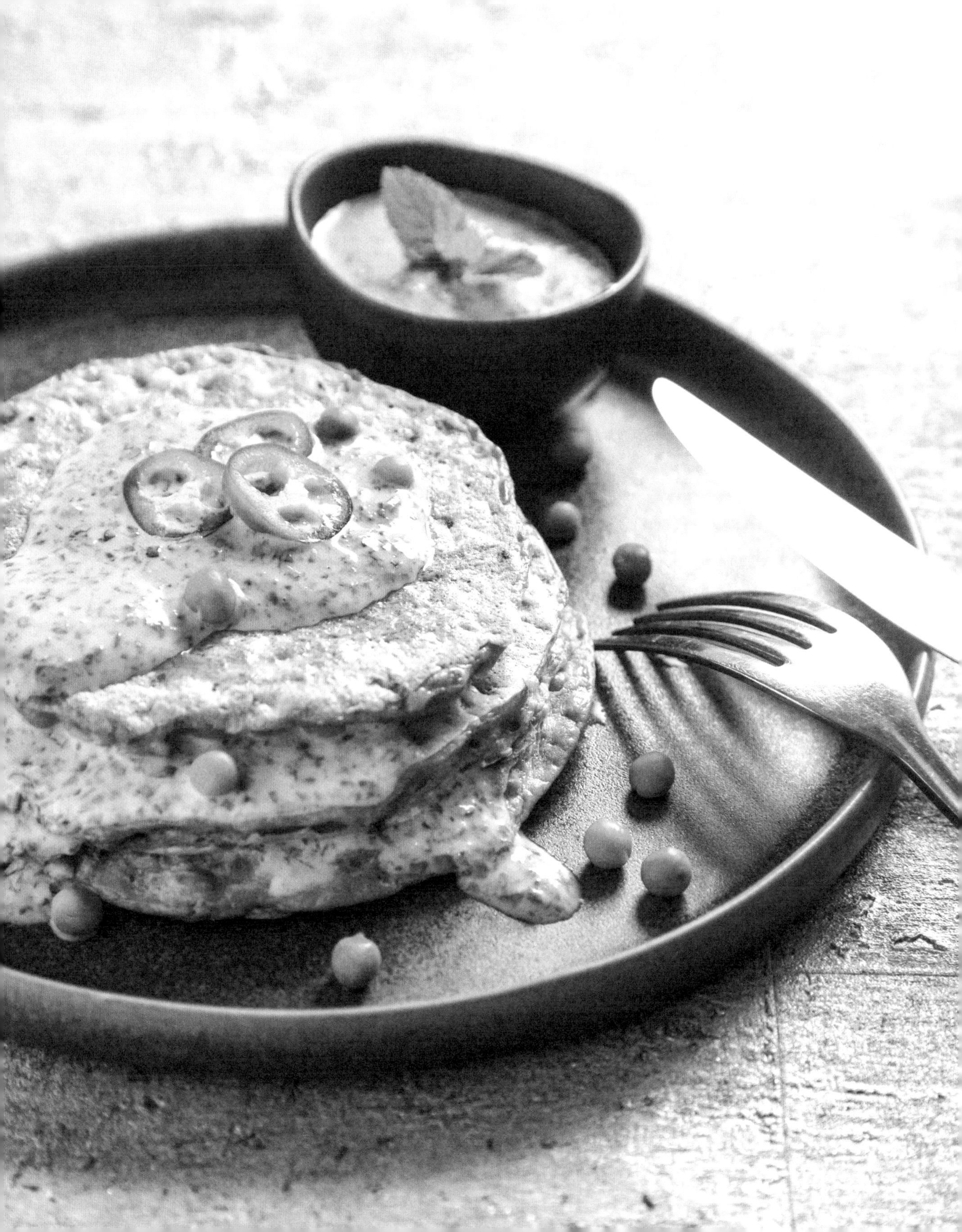

SUPER BRUNCH

SERVES ONE

- 1 plum tomato, cut in half
- ½ tsp dried thyme
- freshly ground black pepper
- firm tofu, the size and thickness of your palm
- ½ tsp turmeric
- ½ tsp paprika
- small pinch of chilli flakes
- small handful of roughly chopped spinach
- small handful of chopped chives (keep 2 whole to garnish)
- ½ tsp white pepper
- ½ avocado

Super Brunch is your secret weapon to feeling supercharged all day. Packed with superfoods like spinach and avocado, it's a great go-to when you have a busy schedule. Loaded with vitamins, antioxidants, and healthy fats, combined with protein-rich tofu, it's as nutritious as it is delicious!

1. Season the tomato with dried thyme and a good grind of black pepper and place under a medium grill.
2. In a pan, crumble the tofu, add the spices and a tablespoon of water, place over a medium heat and stir until hot (about 3 minutes). Now add the spinach and chopped chives and cook for a further minute. Season with white pepper.
3. Once the tomato is juicy and has a nice golden colour, remove from the grill.
4. With a small knife, slice the avocado into a fan shape and place on your plate, add the grilled tomato, spoon on the scrambled tofu, and garnish with the uncut chives.

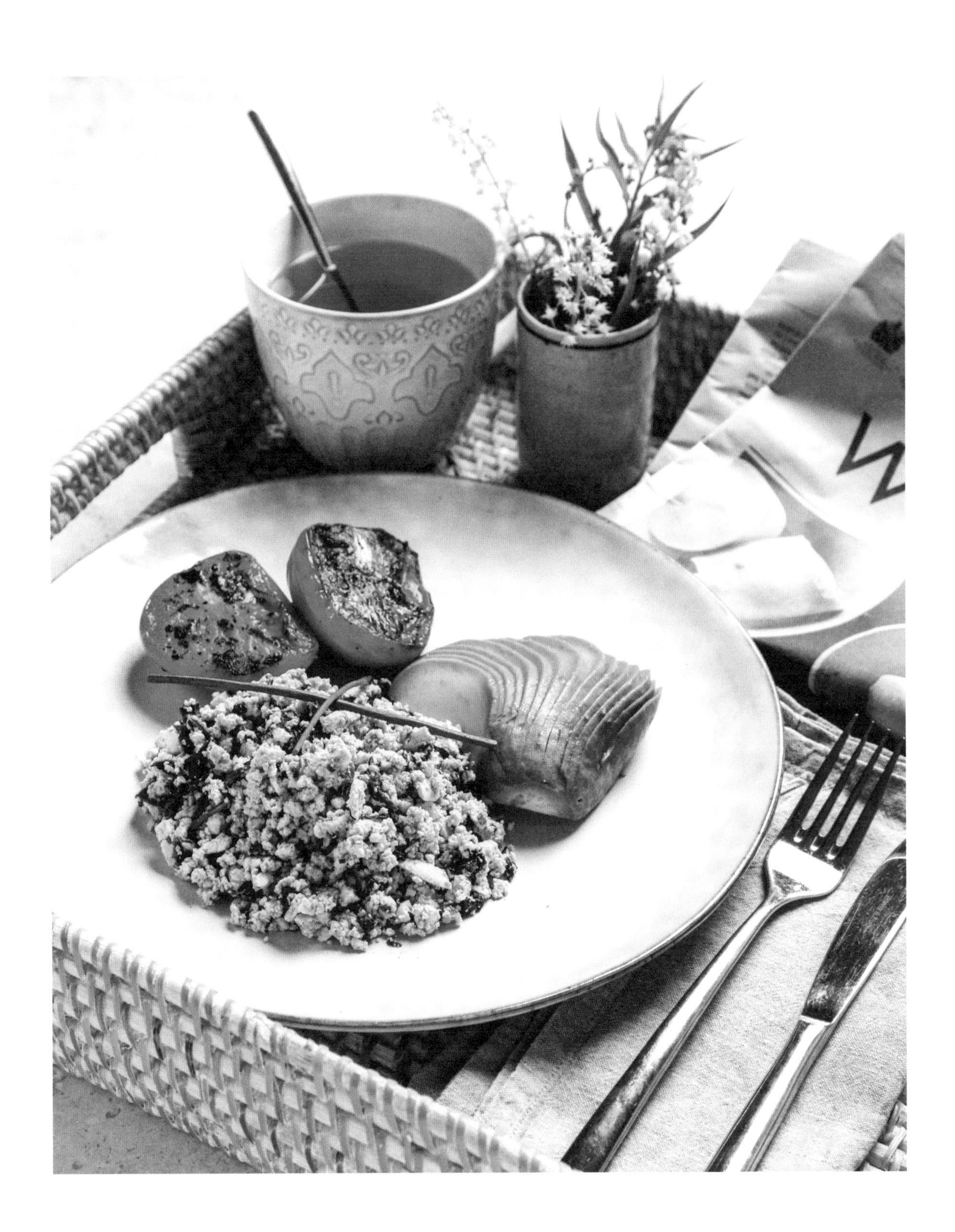

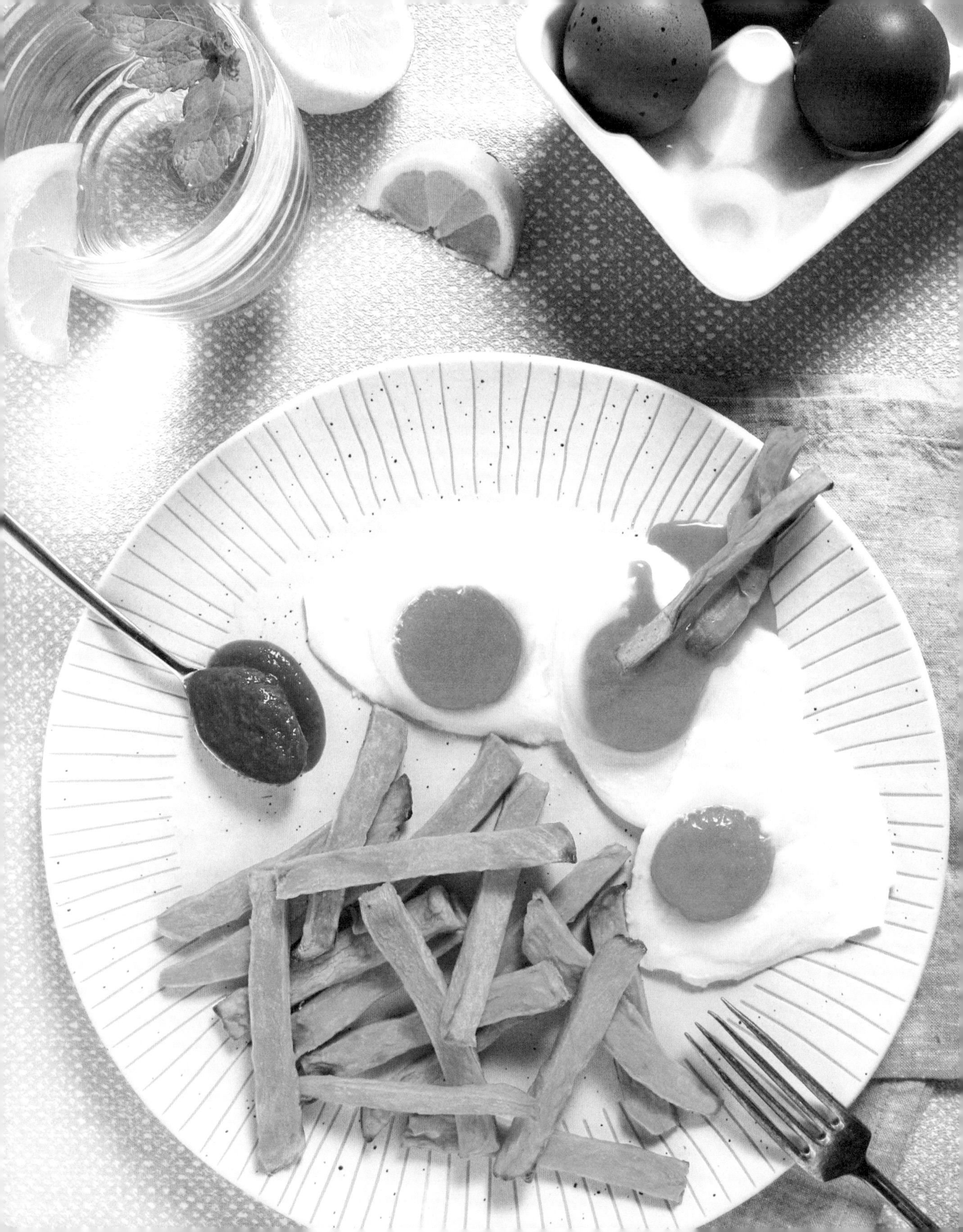

FRIED EGG, CHIPS AND KETCHUP

SERVES ONE

- handful of sweet potato, peeled and cut into chips
- 1 tsp olive oil
- freshly ground black pepper to season (optional)
- 3 eggs

FOR THE KETCHUP

- 1 tbsp tomato paste
- 2 large pinches of white pepper
- ¼ tsp paprika
- juice of ¼ lemon
- freshly ground black pepper

Dive headfirst into this quintessential British treat. It embodies the simple, satisfying classic, yet skips the grease and goes straight for your health in a heartbeat. The eggs and sweet potato are a heart-healthy food choice, packed with nutrients to support cardiovascular wellness. "Frying" the eggs in water is healthier than using fat.

1. Preheat the oven to 180°C (160°C fan/350°F/Gas 4).
2. On a baking tray, toss the sweet potato chips in the olive oil, making sure they are coated, and season with black pepper (if using).
3. Place the baking tray in the oven and cook the chips for 15–20 minutes until lightly browned.
4. While the chips are cooking, make the tomato ketchup. Place all the ingredients in a small bowl with 4 tablespoons of water and stir until thoroughly combined.
5. To cook the eggs, add some water to the bottom of a frying pan to a depth of about 2.5cm (1in) and bring it to the boil. Add the eggs, turn the heat down slightly and "fry" them in the water until cooked to your liking.
6. Serve the eggs and chips on a plate, season with black pepper, and add ketchup, if liked.

GOOD TO KNOW

Put the ketchup in an airtight container and it will last in the fridge for a few days or, alternatively, you can freeze it in a couple of separate freezer bags and it will last a month.

SMOKED SALMON WITH SWEET MELON AND MINT

SERVES ONE

- small handful of cantaloupe melon, cut into small pieces
- 2 slices smoked salmon, chopped
- 3 cherry tomatoes, quartered
- ½ tsp extra virgin olive oil
- juice of ½ lime
- freshly ground black pepper
- 1 tsp fresh chopped mint (reserve a sprig to garnish)

Melon is often served with Parma ham, but I prefer the silkiness of smoked salmon for this refreshing dish. With the addition of aromatic mint, the flavours of the three ingredients work surprisingly well together. You must try this one!

1 Add all the ingredients to a bowl, toss together, season with black pepper, and top with the sprig of fresh mint.

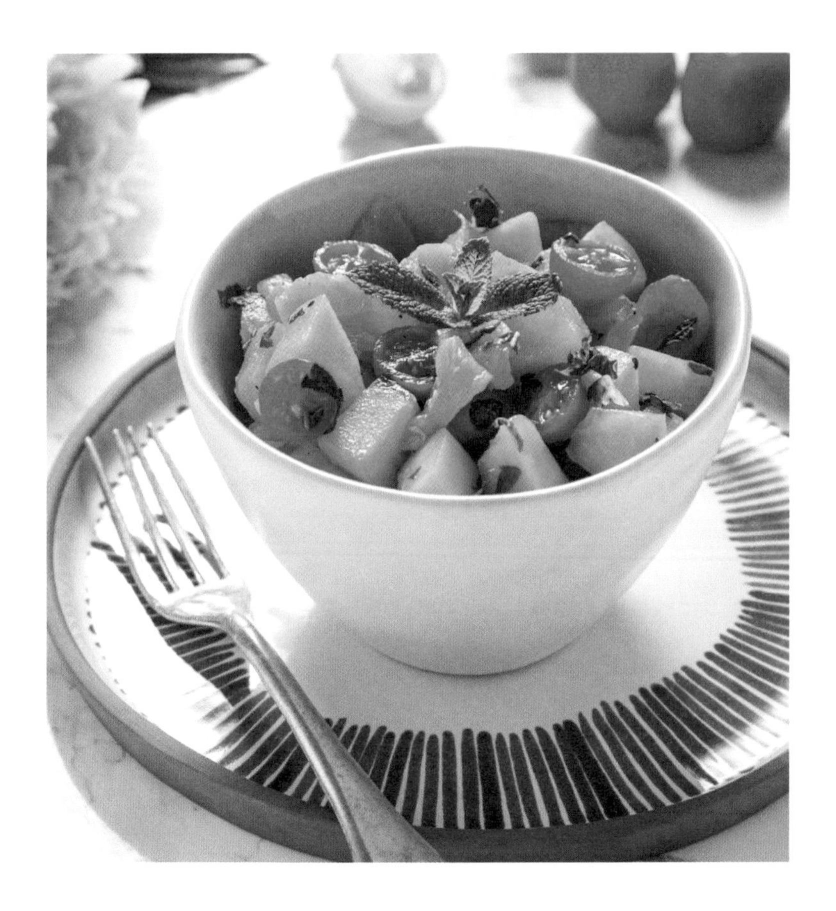

CHUNKY MONKEY CAKE

SERVES FOUR

large handful of ripe banana

45g (generous ⅓ cup) oats

3 scoops of The Six Pack Revolution Decadent Chocolate Caramel Post Workout Protein Shake Powder

1 flat tsp baking powder

100ml (6½ tbsp) unsweetened almond milk

60g (2oz) unsalted roasted peanuts (reserve some for sprinkling on top)

FOR THE TOPPING

1 heaped tbsp full-fat Greek yogurt OR Greek-style soya (soy)-based vegan yogurt

1 tsp The Six Pack Revolution Decadent Chocolate Caramel Post Protein Shake Powder

some of the unsalted roasted peanuts, crushed

Enjoy the taste of days gone by with our Chunky Monkey Cake, inspired by the iconic ice cream flavour that combines chocolate, banana, and nuts. Indulge in memories with every delightful bite, guilt-free, as it's packed with health benefits.

1. Preheat the oven to 180°C (160°C fan/350°F/Gas 4).

2. Mash the banana to a wet consistency and add to a mixing bowl with the oats, protein powder, baking powder, and almond milk and mix thoroughly.

3. Pour the cake mixture into a small, parchment-lined loaf tin and bake in the oven for 30 minutes until cooked through (test with a skewer). Remove from the oven and move to a wire rack to cool. Leave the cake in the tin for a few minutes then turn it out and place on a wire rack to cool completely.

4. To serve, mix the yogurt with the protein powder and spread over to the top of the cake with the back of a spoon. Sprinkle the crushed peanuts on top. Serve cut into slices.

APPLE AND BLACKBERRY MUESLI CAKE

SERVES TWO

- 200ml (scant 1 cup) unsweetened soya (soy) OR unsweetened pea milk
- 1 apple, peeled and chopped into small cubes
- 1 cinnamon stick
- 3 cardamom pods, bashed
- 3 cloves
- 3 tbsp oats
- 1 egg, lightly beaten
- 1 vanilla pod
- 6 blackberries, halved
- 6 pecans, halved
- 3 tbsp full-fat Greek yogurt OR Greek-style soya (soy)-based vegan yogurt

This recipe has a Christmassy feel with its warming spices, sweet berries and its cake-like texture. This is a great healthy alternative to satisfy those cake cravings.

1. Preheat the oven to 180°C (160°C fan/350°F/Gas 4).
2. Add the milk, apple, and all the spices to a pan and bring to the boil. Turn the heat down, cover, and simmer for 10 minutes, then set to one side.
3. In a separate bowl, mix the oats, egg, vanilla seeds (scrape these out of the middle of the pod by scoring then scraping with a knife), blackberries, and pecans.
4. Now remove the spices from the apple and milk, then mash the apple a little with a fork. Pour this into the oat mixture, stir, and transfer to a small ovenproof dish.
5. Cook in the oven for 30 minutes and serve straight from the dish topped with the yogurt.

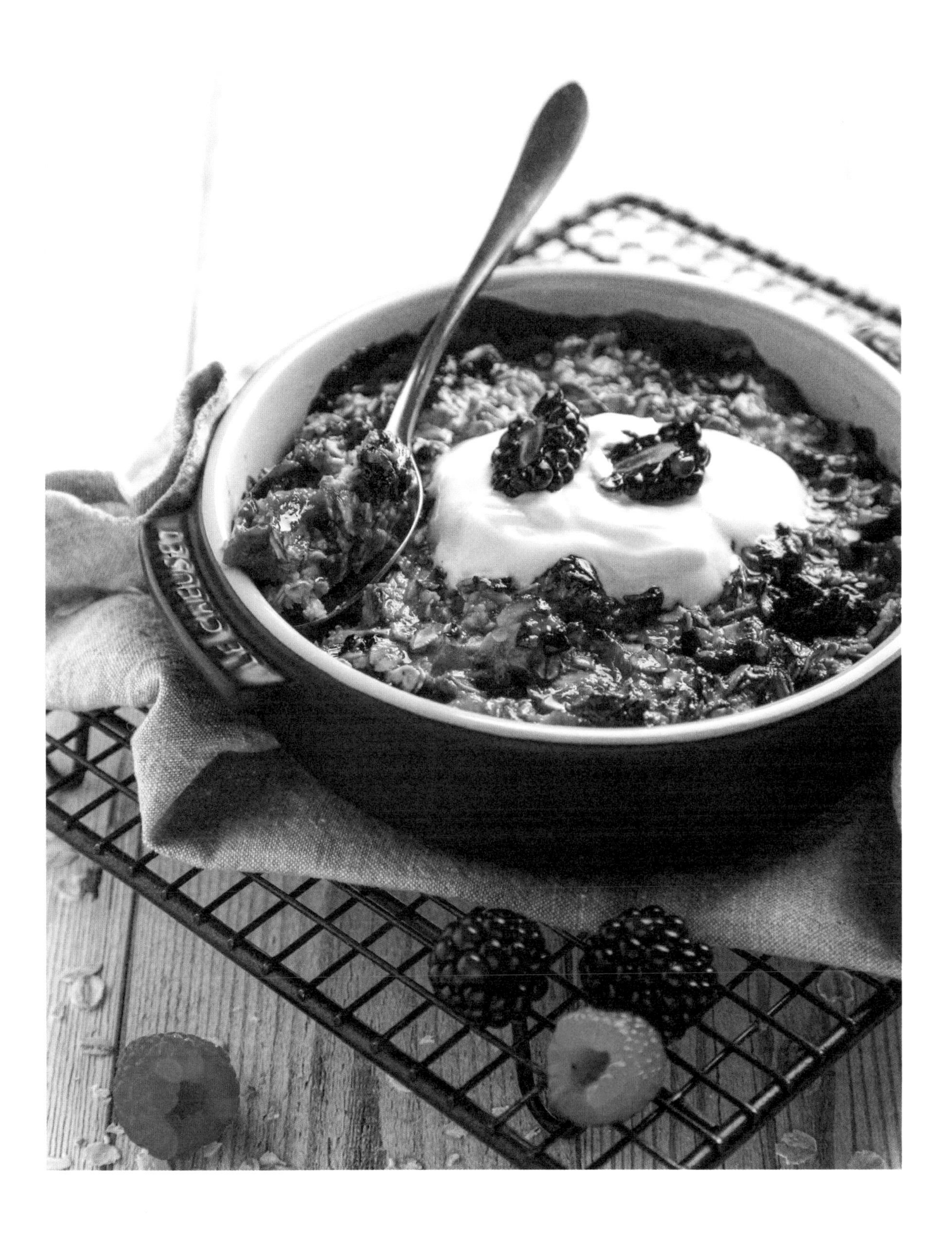

CARROT CAKE

SERVES FOUR

- 1 medium carrot, grated
- large handful of ripe banana, mashed
- 60g (2oz) walnut halves (reserve some for the topping)
- 3 scoops of The Six Pack Revolution Vanilla Caramel Heaven Post Workout Protein Shake Powder
- 45g (⅓ cup) oats
- 100ml (6½ tbsp) unsweetened almond milk
- 1 flat tsp baking powder
- ½ tsp cinnamon

FOR THE TOPPING

- 1 heaped tbsp full-fat Greek yogurt OR Greek-style soya (soy)-based vegan yogurt
- sprinkle of walnuts

Did someone say cake? Oh yes, we have cake and it's healthy! Gather around, share with friends, savour with a black coffee. It's time to indulge guilt-free.

1. Preheat the oven to 180°C (160°C fan/350°F/Gas 4).
2. Crush the walnuts by placing them in a clear bag and bashing with a rolling pin until they are in small pieces.
3. Add all the ingredients except for the topping to a mixing bowl, combine thoroughly and pour into a baking parchment-lined loaf tin.
4. Place in the oven for 30 minutes or until cooked through.
5. Remove the cake from the oven then leave to cool slightly in the tin, before turning out onto a wire rack to cool completely.
6. To make the topping, spread the yogurt over the top of the cake with the back of a spoon and scatter over the remaining crushed walnuts.

GOOD TO KNOW

You can store the cake without the Greek yogurt topping for a few days in an airtight container.

LEMON, BLUEBERRY, AND POPPY SEED DRIZZLE CAKE

SERVES FOUR

- 75g (½ cup) oats
- juice and zest of 1½ lemons
- 3 scoops of The Six Pack Revolution Vanilla Caramel Heaven Post Workout Protein Shake Powder
- small handful of blueberries
- 1 flat tsp baking powder
- 2 tbsp poppy seeds (reserve some for sprinkling on top)
- 200ml (scant 1 cup) unsweetened almond milk

FOR THE TOPPING

- 1 heaped tbsp full-fat Greek yogurt OR Greek-style soya (soy)-based vegan yogurt
- sprinkle of poppy seeds

A blueberry and poppy seed muffin reimagined in cake form with a healthy twist! Packed with protein goodness from our very own protein powder, it's a treat you can savour without the sugar overload.

1. Preheat the oven to 180°C (160°C fan/350°F/Gas 4).
2. Add the oats, all the lemon juice, half the zest of one lemon, protein powder, blueberries, baking powder, and almond milk and mix thoroughly.
3. Pour the mixture into a small baking parchment-lined loaf tin and put it in the oven for 30 minutes.
4. Remove the cake from the oven and move to a wire rack, then squeeze the juice of the remaining half lemon over the top and leave to cool.
5. To serve, top with the yogurt, a sprinkle of poppy seeds, and the zest of half a lemon.

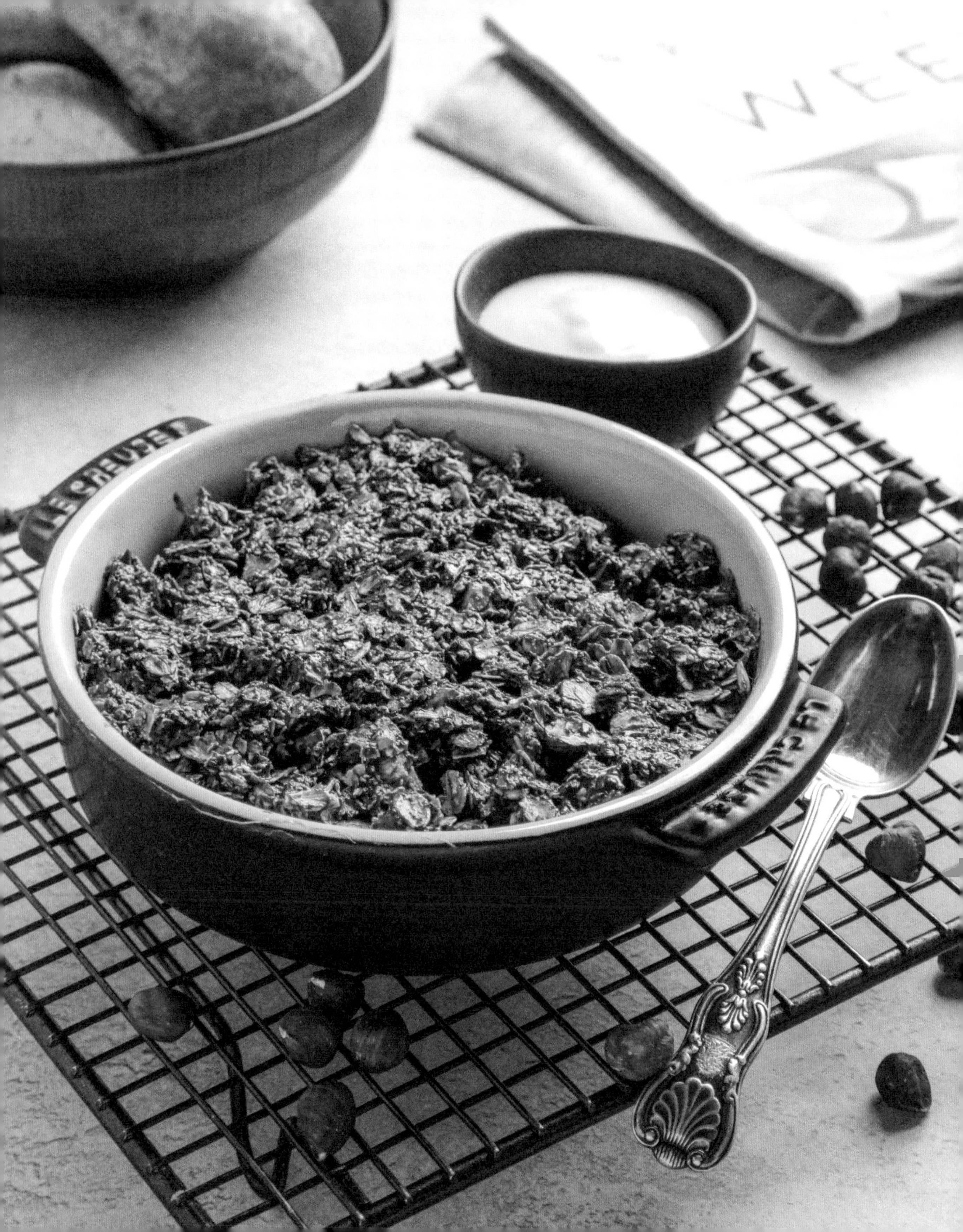
LE CREUSET

CHOCOLATE AND PEAR CRUMBLE

SERVES TWO

- 1 pear, peeled and chopped
- 3 tbsp whole rolled oats
- ½ serving of The Six Pack Revolution Decadent Chocolate Caramel Post Workout Protein Shake Powder
- 6 hazelnuts, roughly chopped
- juice of 1 lemon
- 3 tbsp full-fat Greek yogurt OR Greek-style soya (soy)-based vegan yogurt

Who doesn't love a crumble? This decadent, rich in flavour version warms you up and comes with a delicious crunchy hat!

1. Preheat the oven to 180°C (160°C fan/350°F/Gas 4).
2. Cover the bottom of a small ovenproof dish with the pear.
3. Put the oats, the protein powder, hazelnuts, and lemon juice in a bowl and mix with your fingers until you have a sticky texture.
4. Add the crumble mixture on top of the pear in the ovenproof dish, place in the oven, and cook for 20 minutes.
5. If you want to make the topping more golden, place the dish under a medium hot grill (broiler) for a few minutes.
6. Serve in a bowl with the yogurt.

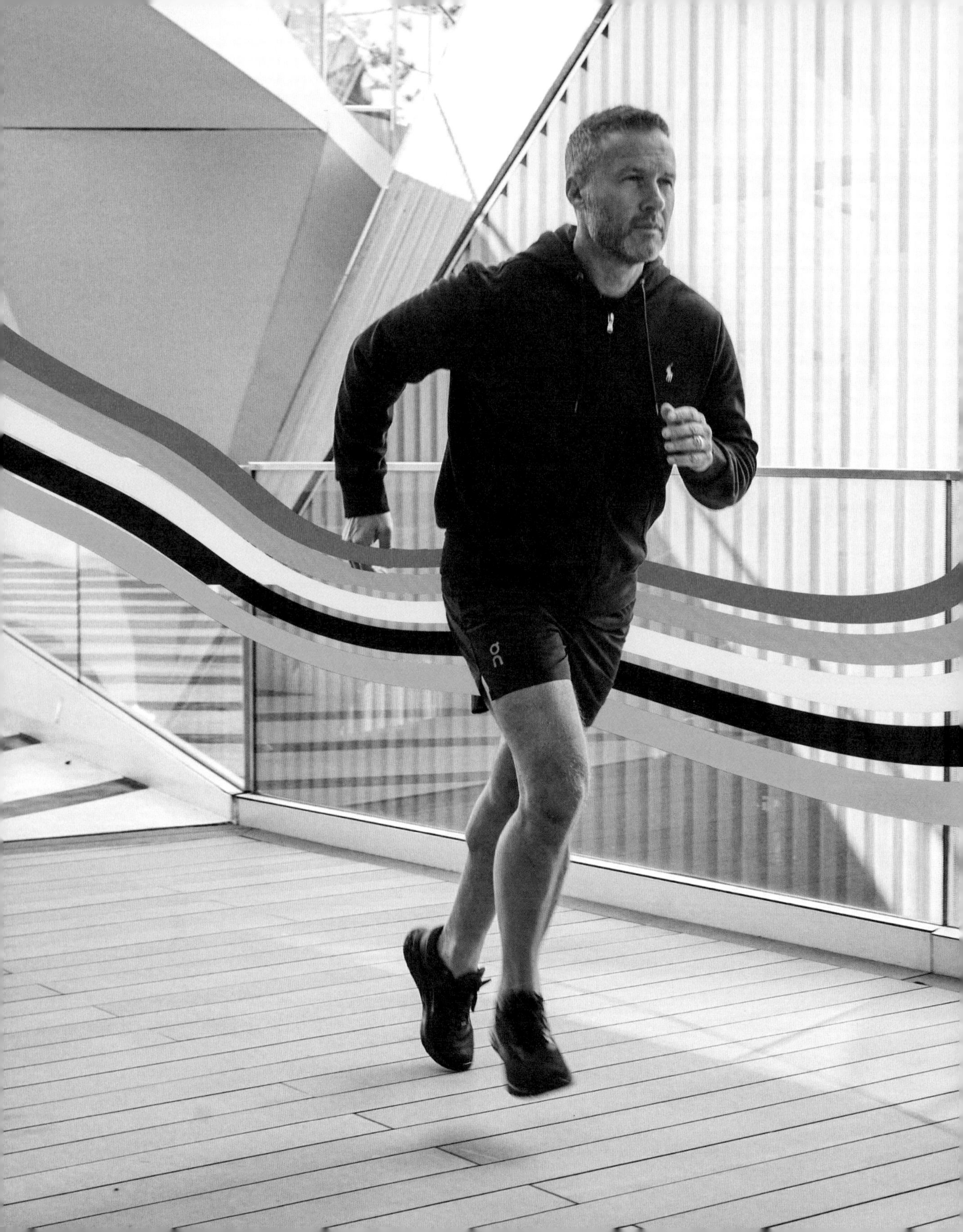

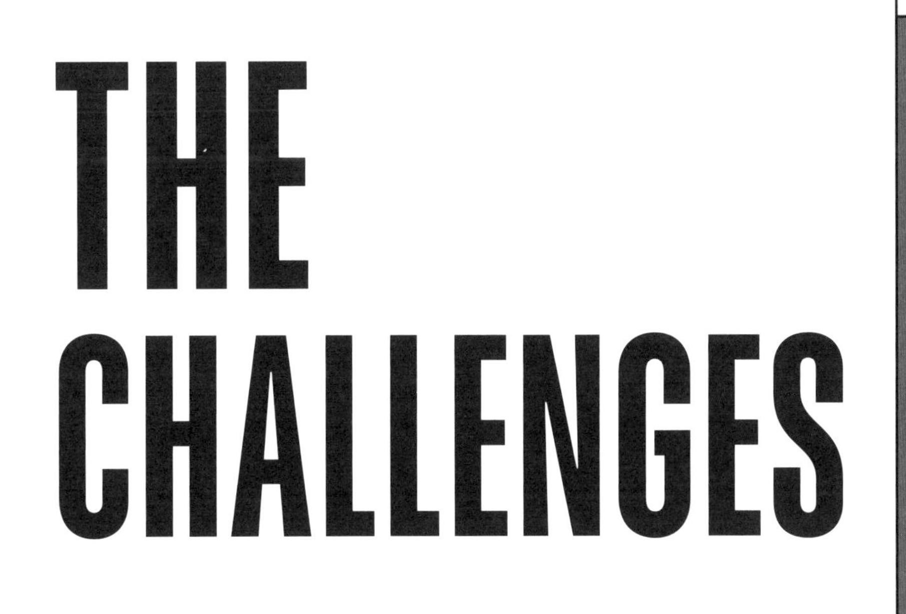

THE CHALLENGES

Chapter 3

NOW LET'S GO TO WORK

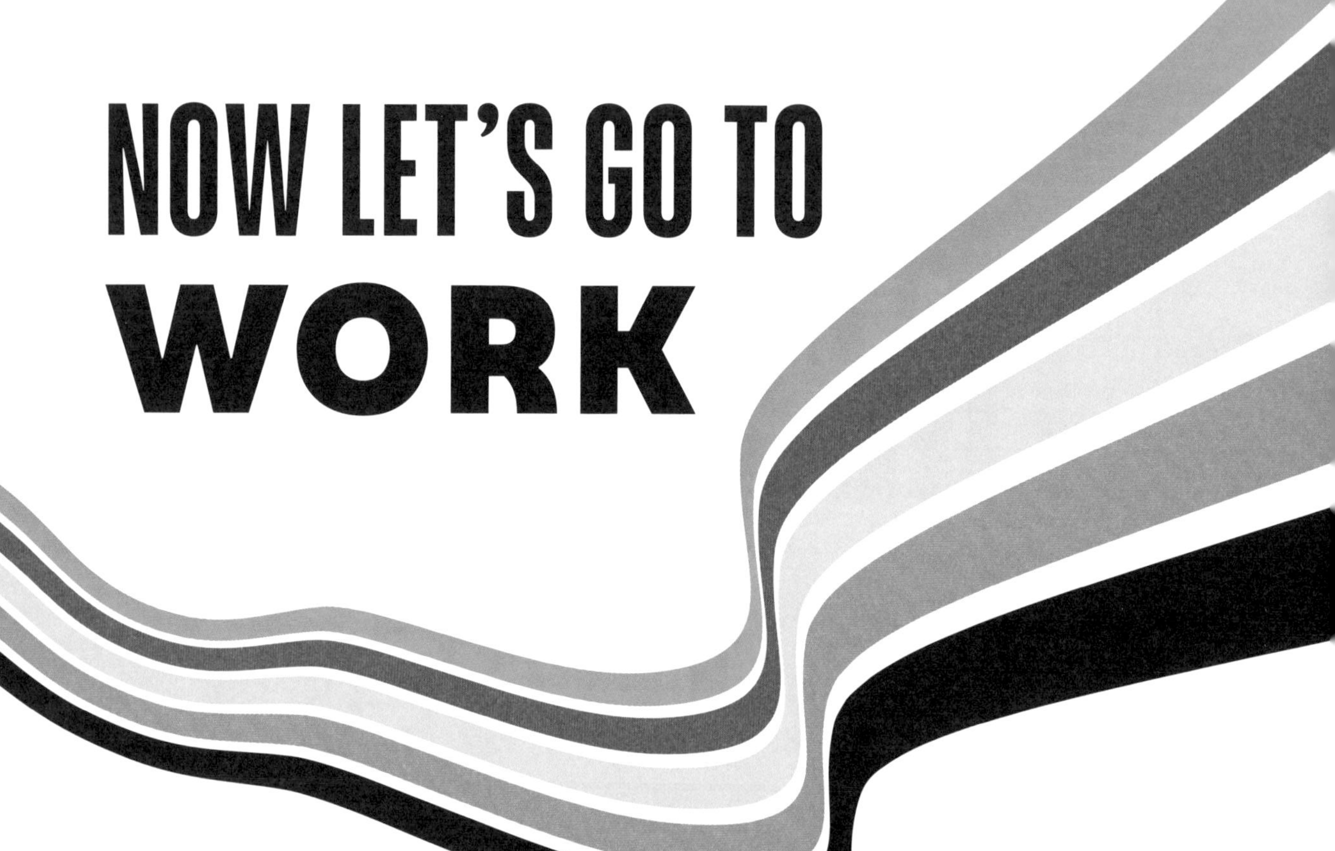

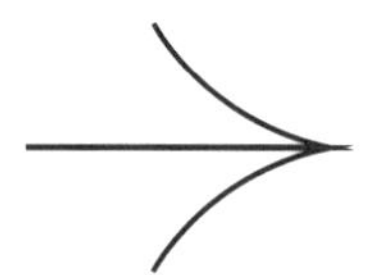

Kettlebells provide high-intensity, full-body movements, which help to increase calorie expenditure and boost metabolism, promoting fat loss. Additionally, the muscular engagement from kettlebell exercises helps preserve lean muscle mass, crucial for maintaining a healthy metabolism. Every workout can be done indoors, so you can get to work even if it's raining hard outside, and on a nice day you can rock the bells alfresco!

THE BENEFITS OF KETTLEBELL TRAINING

- **Low-impact cardiovascular fitness**
- **Full-body strength building**
- **Boosts coordination and mobility**
- **Fights imbalances and asymmetries**
- **Easy to master**
- **Efficient calorie burn**

If you're new to kettlebells you'll want to choose a kettlebell based on your current abilities and fitness levels, and for the selected exercise. For example, you may be able to deadlift 16kg (35lb) but may not be able to lift it overhead for a halo or overhead press. Your kettlebell shouldn't be so light that you can swing it too fast or lift it with ease, however, avoid a kettlebell that is so heavy you can barely lift it.

Remember, you will be lifting and swinging a weight so make sure you have enough room and are clear of any obstacles.

Take a break at any time between sets or after a complete round. Work to your own ability but push yourself – the only person you need to challenge is YOU! And remember to do your warm-up routine before you jump into the kettlebell circuit.

Each of these workouts can be used to squeeze a quick 10 minute session into a busy day, repeat for the recommended 2 or 3 rounds for a longer workout, or you could even pick 2 or 3 different routines to perform back-to-back to for an intense all over body blast.

“ REGRET DOESN’T COME FROM COMMITTING TO SOMETHING AND MESSING UP. TRUE REGRET COMES FROM NEVER COMMITTING TO ANYTHING AT ALL.”

SCOTT HARRISON

YOUR WARM UP IS IMPORTANT

You need to make sure you warm up, momentum forms the main part of most kettlebell routines so a warm up is essential. Get your body ready by following our full body warm up to get the heart pumping and blood flowing to power your workout.

TAKE CARE OF YOUR BACK

Choose a kettlebell weight that challenges you but is not too heavy so it allows you to maintain good form. Form wins over weight every time.

BREATHE

Make sure you're breathing through the exercises, exhale on the effort, inhale on the return. This will help you to use your breathing technique to engage your abs which in turn will keep your back in alignment and help protect the spine.

BE AWARE

Make sure you are aware of your surroundings when swinging your kettlebell. Allow yourself space from other people. Make sure your exercise area is clear and there are no obstacles in the way of your swing area. Also, be aware that different kettlebell weights will be needed for different exercises.

WARM UP

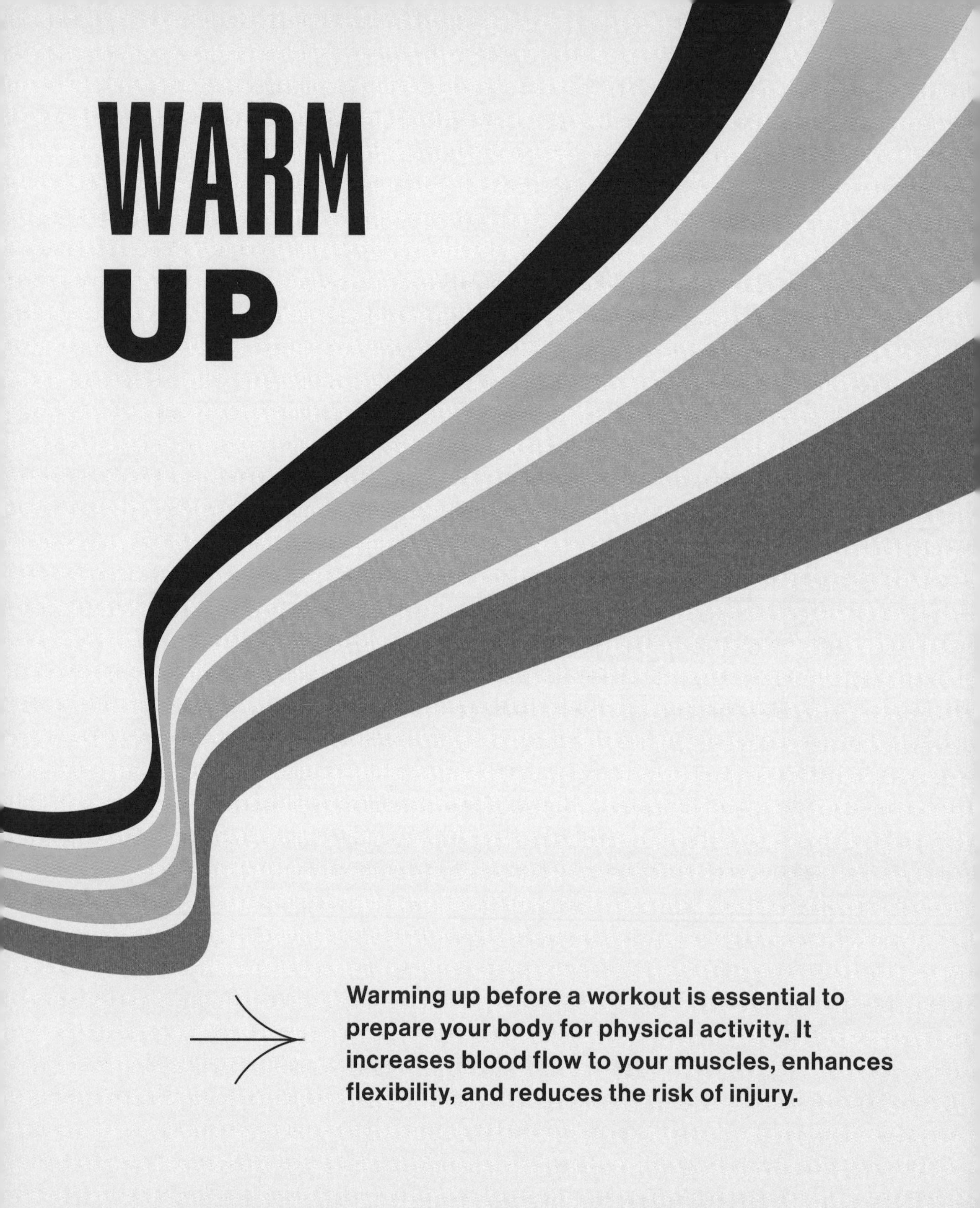

Warming up before a workout is essential to prepare your body for physical activity. It increases blood flow to your muscles, enhances flexibility, and reduces the risk of injury.

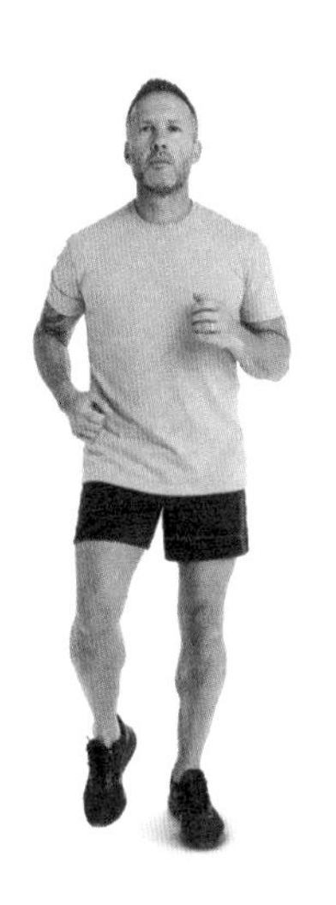

LOW LEVEL JOG

30 seconds

1 Start in a standing position with arms hanging loosely by the sides, come to a light jog on the spot, keeping the shoulders and arms relaxed.

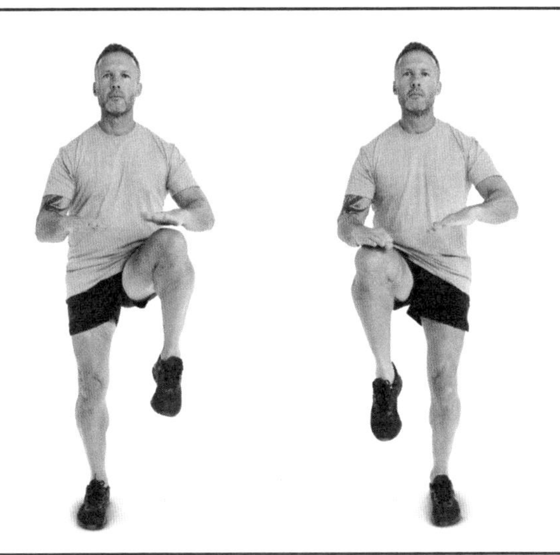

HIGH KNEES

30 seconds

1 From your low level jog, increase the intensity by lifting alternate knees towards the chest at a faster pace. Pick a point to focus your gaze on in front of you to aid your balance. Bend the elbows, holding your hands at waist height as a guide, if you need to. Aim to raise the knee to hand height.

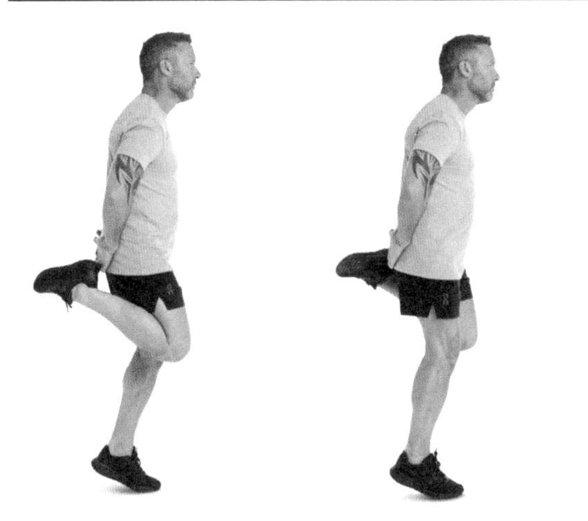

KICK BACKS

30 seconds

1 From your high knees, maintaining the pace, kick your feet alternately back towards your bottom.

FORWARD LUNGES

x 10 on each side

1. Start by standing with feet hip width apart and hands by sides. Take a big step forwards with your left foot and bend at the knee until both knees form 90-degree angles, lowering the body.
2. Press down into your left heel to push back to starting position. Repeat on the right.

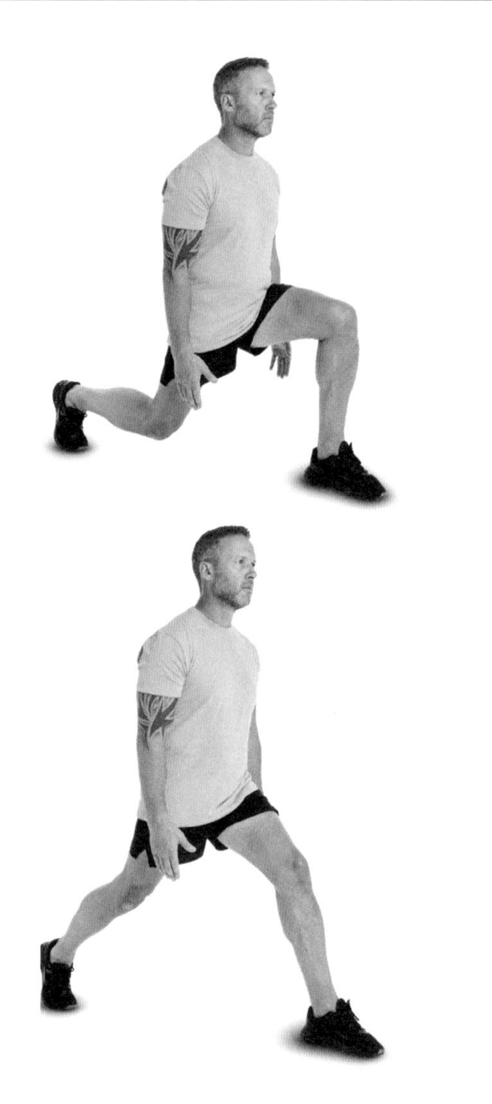

FORWARD LUNGES WITH ROTATION

x 10 on each side

1. Take a big step forwards with your left foot and bend at the knee until both knees form 90 degree angles, lowering the body.
2. Rotate your torso to the left then return to the centre. Press down into your left heel to push back to the starting position. Repeat on the right.

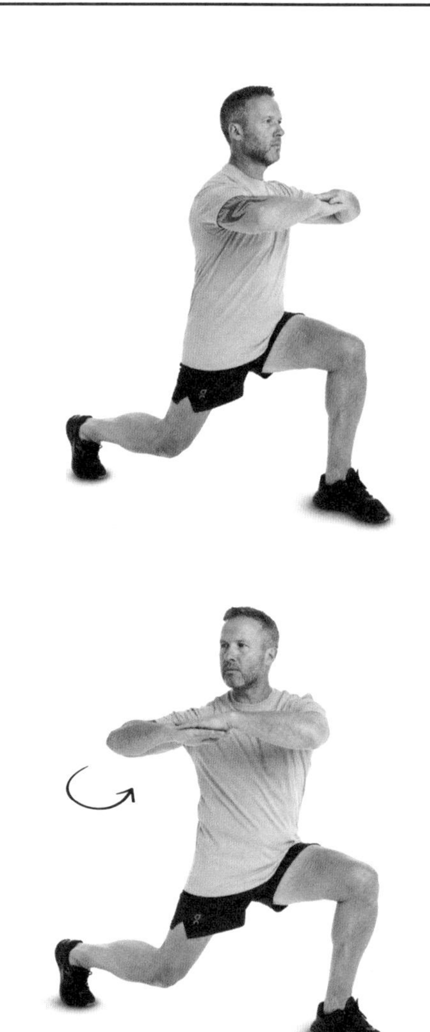

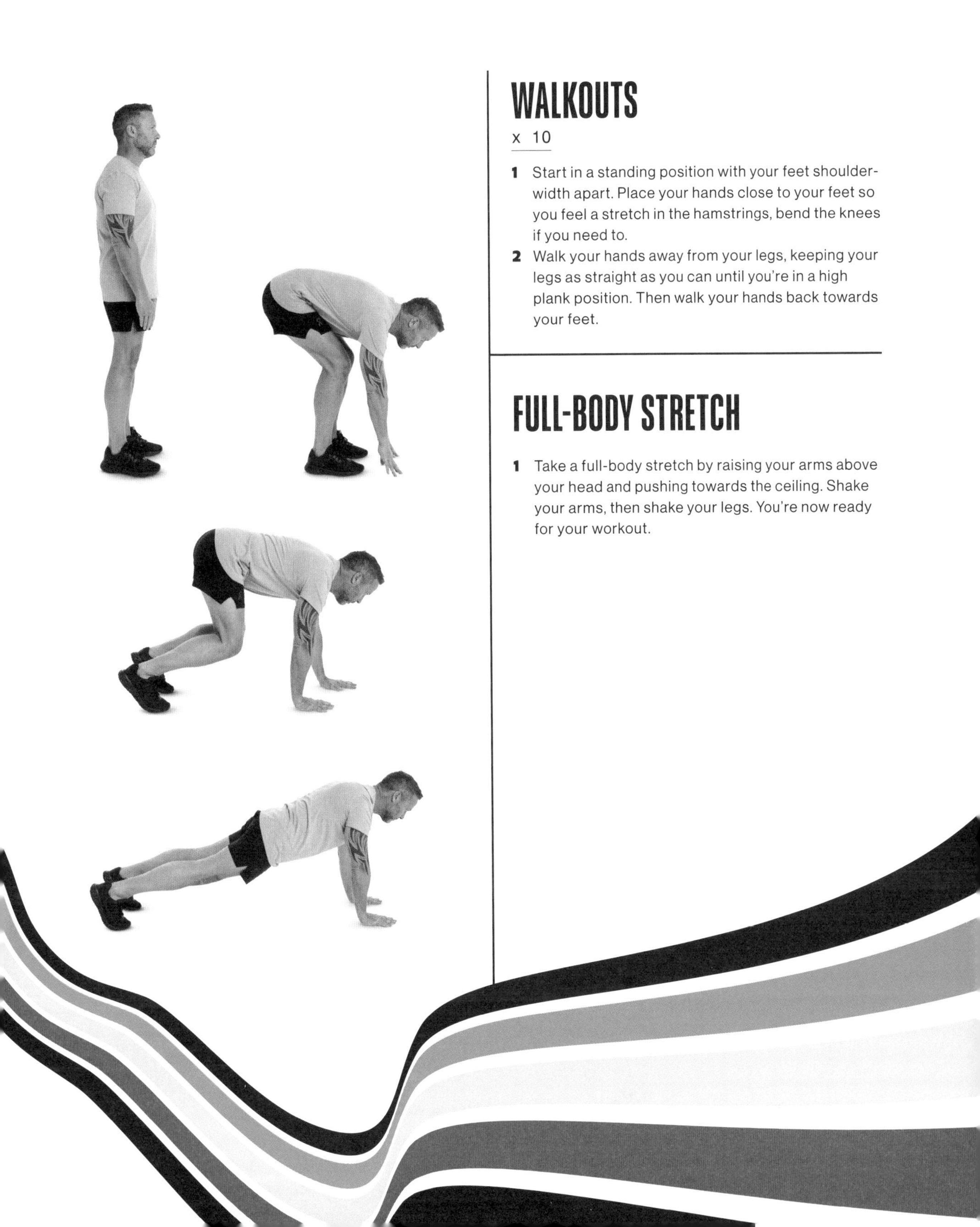

WALKOUTS

x 10

1. Start in a standing position with your feet shoulder-width apart. Place your hands close to your feet so you feel a stretch in the hamstrings, bend the knees if you need to.
2. Walk your hands away from your legs, keeping your legs as straight as you can until you're in a high plank position. Then walk your hands back towards your feet.

FULL-BODY STRETCH

1. Take a full-body stretch by raising your arms above your head and pushing towards the ceiling. Shake your arms, then shake your legs. You're now ready for your workout.

COOL DOWN

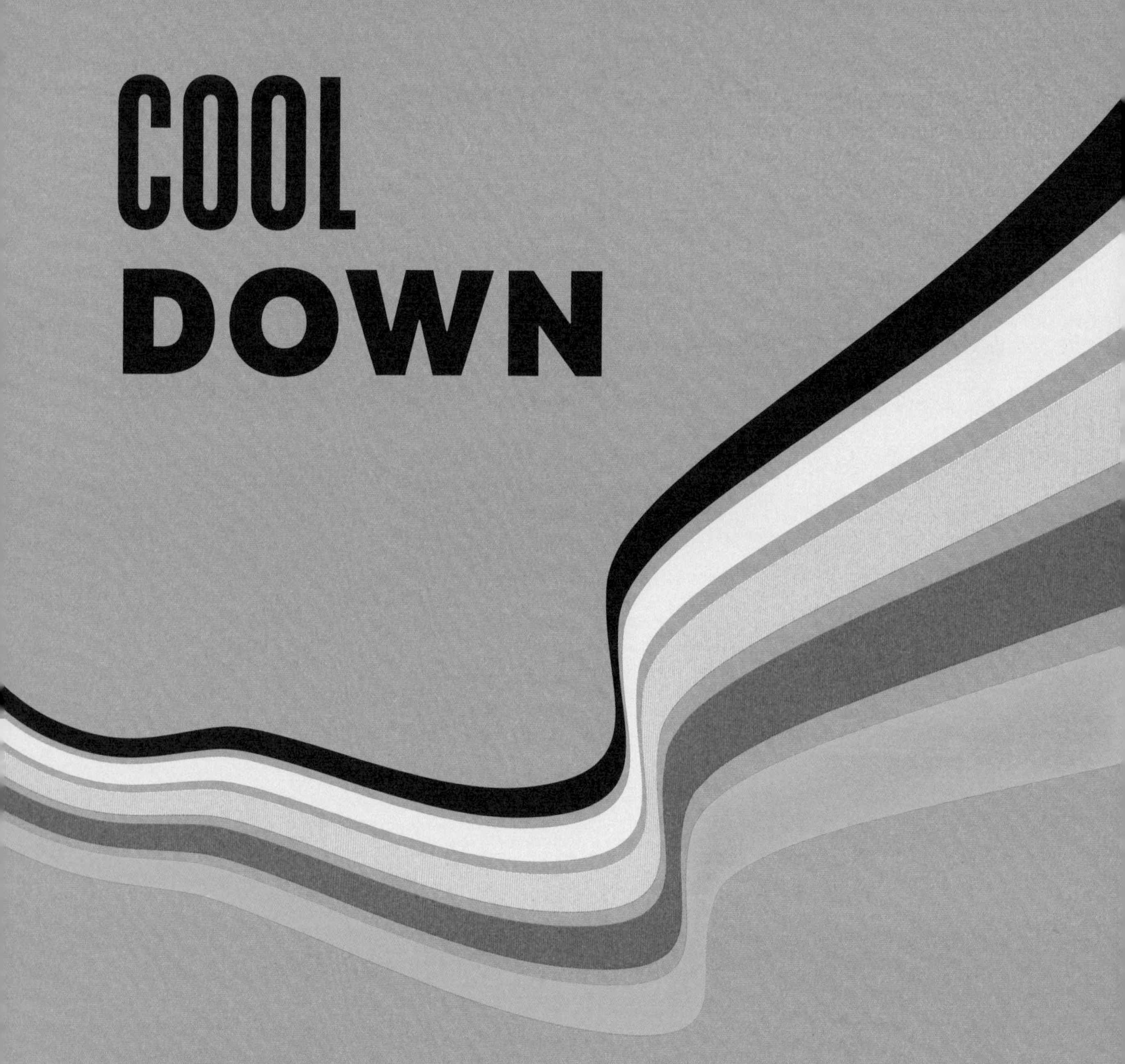

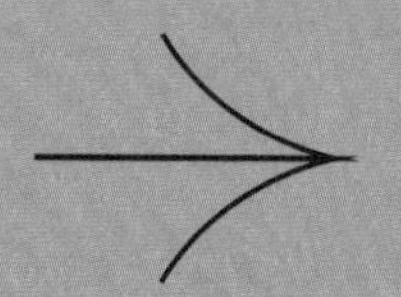

It is important to stretch after EVERY workout to slowly bring your heart rate down and your muscles back to a resting state. This will also help to avoid soreness and injuries and allow you to relax after you've worked hard.

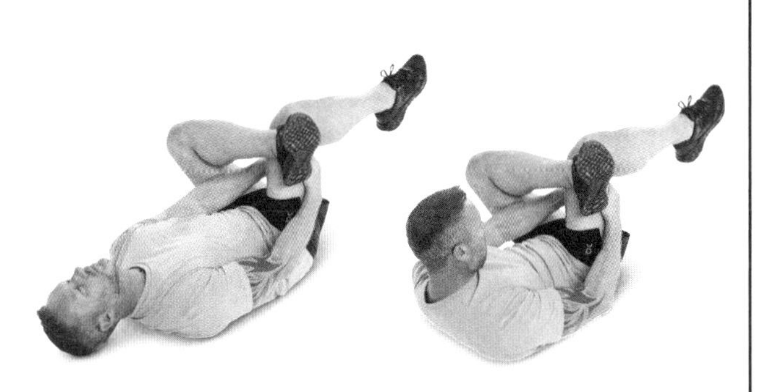

GLUTE STRETCH

Hold for 10 seconds

1 Lie with your back flat on the floor, your arms by your sides, and your knees bent with feet flat on the floor. Raise your right leg and hold your left leg at a right angle to it, holding the right leg underneath with hands clasped. Hold for 10 seconds.
2 To feel the stretch more, lift your head and shoulders, engage your core and pull your left leg closer and tighter. Repeat on the other side.

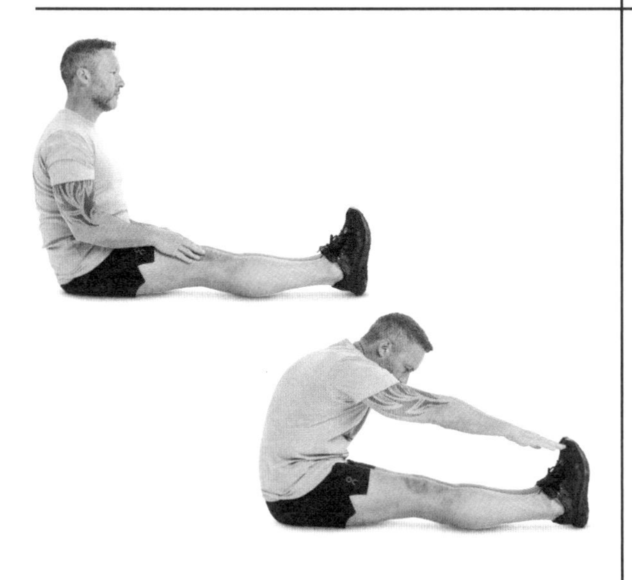

FORWARD BEND / HAMSTRING STRETCH

Hold for 5 seconds

1 Come to a seated position with your legs stretched out in front of you. Take a deep breath in and as you exhale reach towards your toes. Breathe in deeply and reach a little further. Hold for a count of five.
2 If you can touch your toes, great! If not, focus on reaching a little further with each breath.

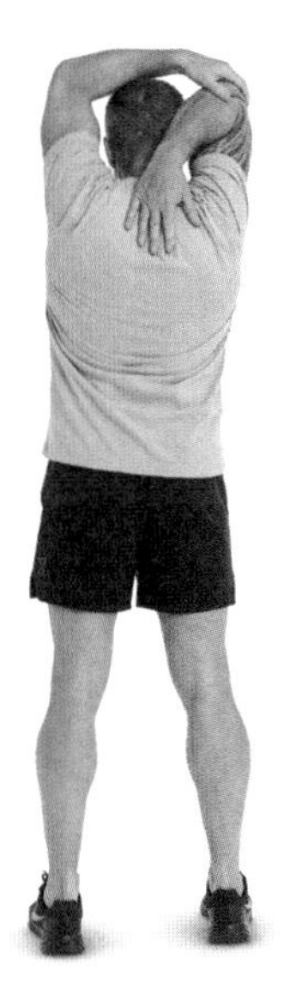

TRICEP STRETCH

Hold for 10 seconds

1 Stand with your feet shoulder-width apart. Take one arm straight up then bend it so the palm of the hand reaches between your shoulder blades, while the elbow stays pointed towards the sky. Place the other hand on the elbow and gently apply pressure to extend the stretch. Hold for 10 seconds. Repeat on the opposite side.

CROSS-ARM STRETCH

Hold for 10 seconds

1 Stand with your feet shoulder-width apart and extend one arm across your body to the opposite side. With the other arm, place the inside of the wrist on the elbow and gently apply pressure to find the stretch. Repeat on the opposite side.

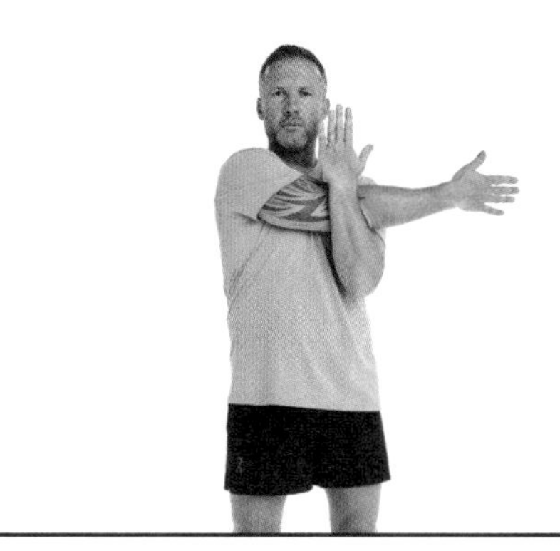

BACK AND CHEST STRETCH

Hold for 5 seconds

1 Stand with your feet shoulder-width apart and straighten your arms out in front of you, interlacing the fingers. Keeping the arms straight, push forwards so you feel the stretch through the upper back and shoulders.
2 Straighten your arms behind you, fingers interlaced. Keeping your arms straight, push backwards, and raise them so you feel the stretch through your chest.

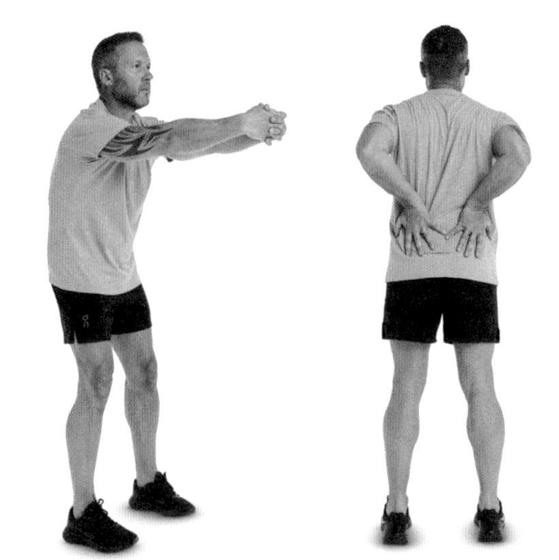

SHAKE DOWN

1 Standing with your feet slightly wider than hip width apart, take a deep breath in while sweeping your arms above your head. Bend your knees slightly and sweep your arms back down as you exhale. And repeat.
2 Shake your arms, shake your legs and bring your hands together in front of your chest.

FULL BODY STRETCH

Hold for 10 seconds

1 Lay on the floor with legs outstretched and arms by your sides. Take your right arm over your head and towards the floor so your elbow is in line with your ear. Stretch the right arm and left leg away from your centre, hold for the count of 10 and feel the stretch through the body. Return to the start position. Repeat with the left arm and right leg.

Your cool down is now complete.

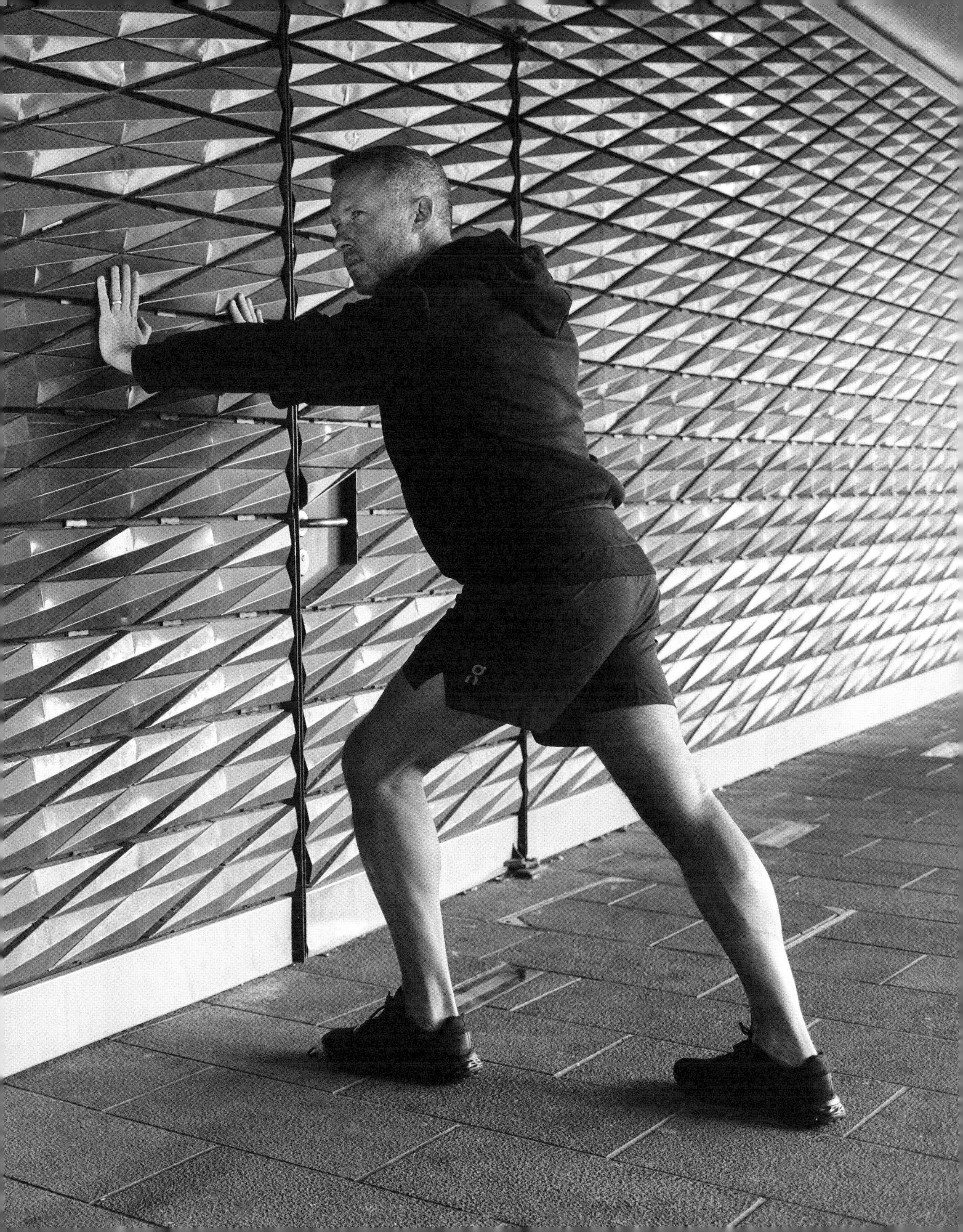

EXERCISE CHALLENGES

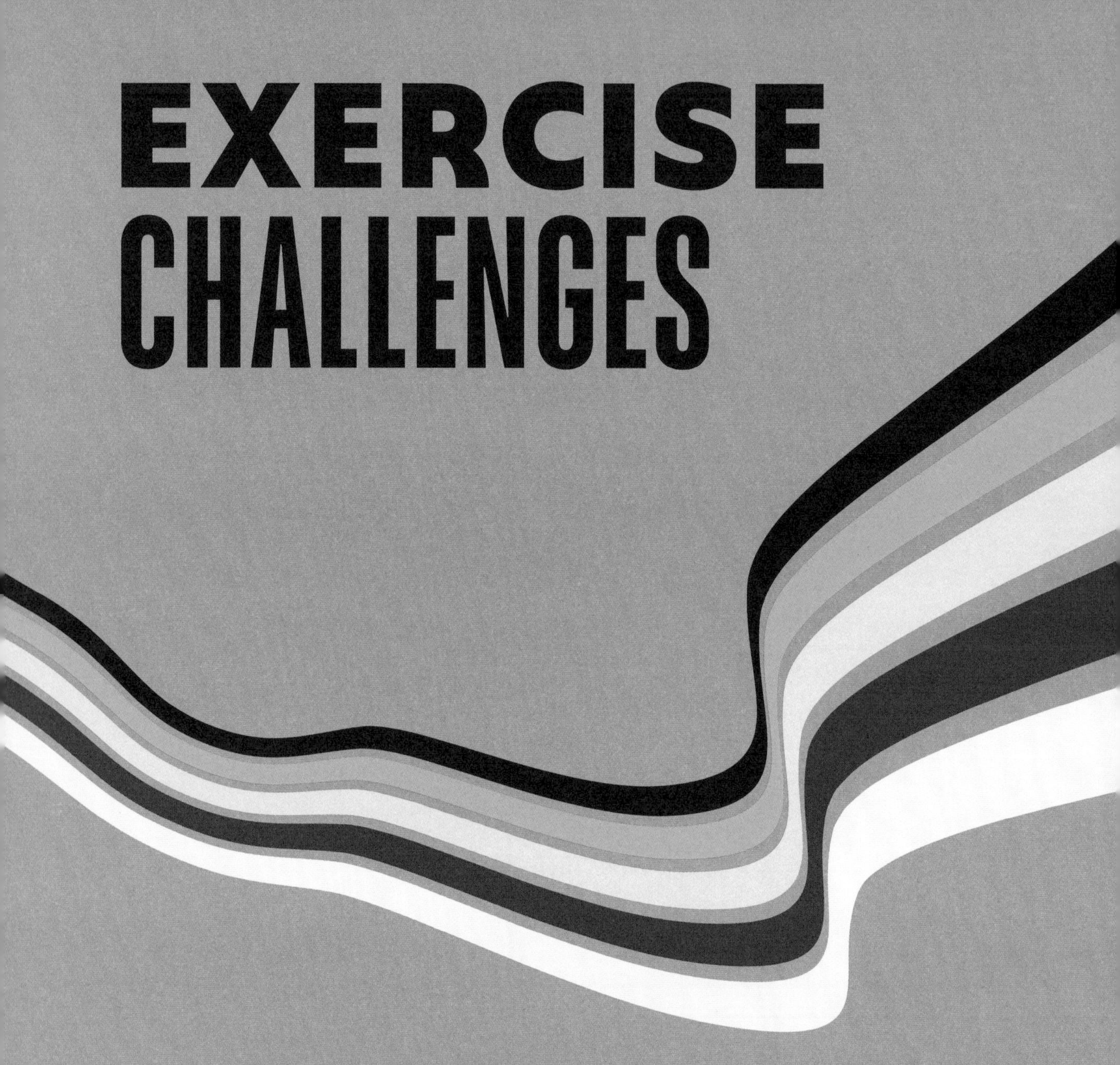

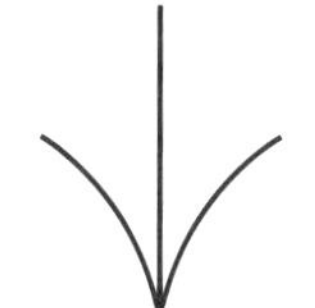

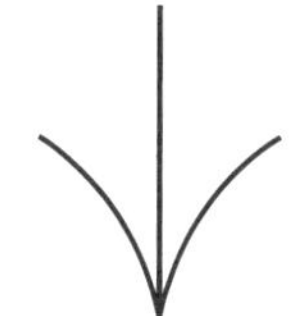

CHALLENGE 1	Get to grips
CHALLENGE 2	Put your back into it
CHALLENGE 3	Twist and shout
CHALLENGE 4	King of the swingers
CHALLENGE 5	Twenty ten time
CHALLENGE 6	Core connection
CHALLENGE 7	Eat, sleep, rep, repeat
CHALLENGE 8	It's all gone sideways
CHALLENGE 9	Ground zero
CHALLENGE 10	Perfectly balanced
CHALLENGE 11	Top and tail

CHALLENGE 1

GET TO GRIPS

- Let's get out of the blocks and master some basic kettlebell moves. This workout uses short bursts of energy to challenge your muscles, increase your heart rate and get used to the feel and movement of the kettlebell.
- Perform each exercise in the sequence 10 times, aim for 15–30 seconds rest between exercises.
- Repeat three times, resting as needed at the end of each round.

KETTLEBELL SWINGS

1. **START POSITION:** Stand with your back straight and feet shoulder-width apart holding the kettlebell with both hands, arms extended.
2. Engage your core, bend your knees as you straighten your legs, push from the heels and explode through the hips, swinging the kettlebell to chest height. As you swing the kettlebell down between your legs, return to the half-squat position and repeat.

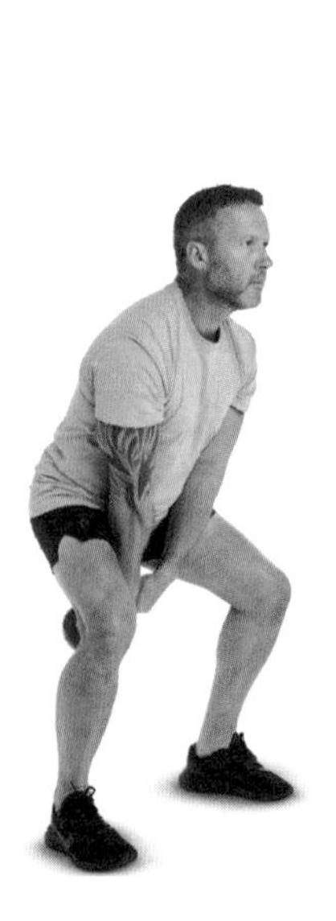

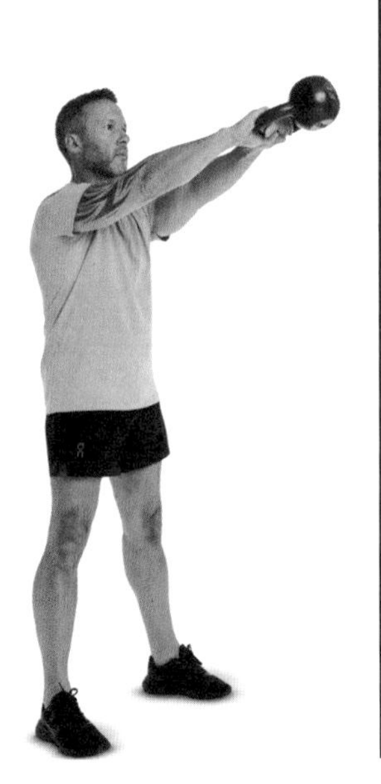

GOBLET SQUATS

1. **START POSITION:** Stand with your feet shoulder-width apart. Hold the kettlebell in front of your chest by the sides of its handle. Tuck your elbows in.
2. Keeping your back straight and core engaged, push your hips back and squat down as if sitting down into a chair. Drive your weight through the heels to push back to a standing position.

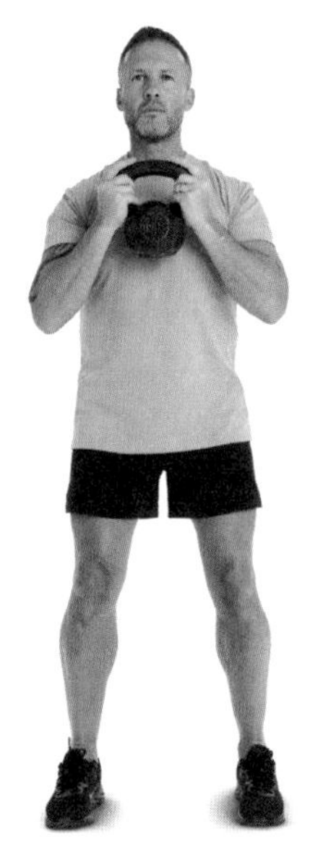

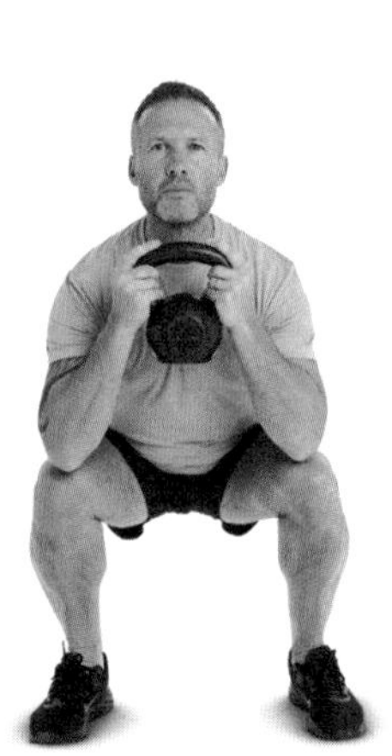

HAND-TO-HAND SWINGS

1 **START POSITION:** Stand with your back straight and feet shoulder-width apart, holding the kettlebell in one hand, arm extended. Engage your core, bend your knees as you straighten your leg push from the heels and explode through the hips, swinging the kettlebell to chest height. Exchange grip from one hand to the other.
2 As you swing the kettlebell down between your legs, return to the half-squat position and repeat, alternating between each hand.

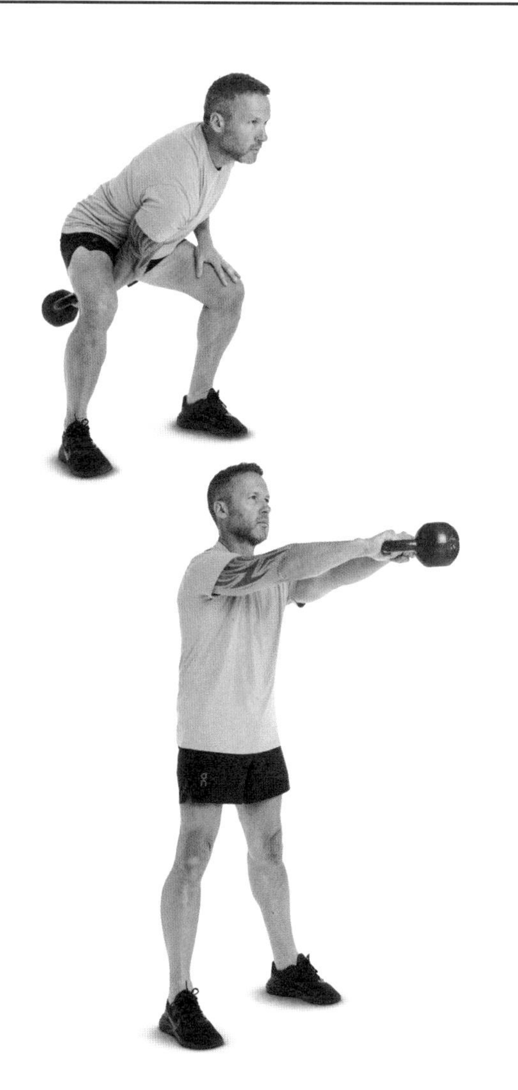

ALTERNATING HALOS

1 **START POSITION:** Stand with your feet shoulder-width apart, holding the kettlebell bottom-up by the horns in front of your chest.
2 Start the movement by aiming the kettlebell over one shoulder like a sandbag. Keeping your eyes forwards with your head and neck still, move the kettlebell steadily around the back of your head to the opposite shoulder until it's back to the starting position. Repeat in the opposite direction.

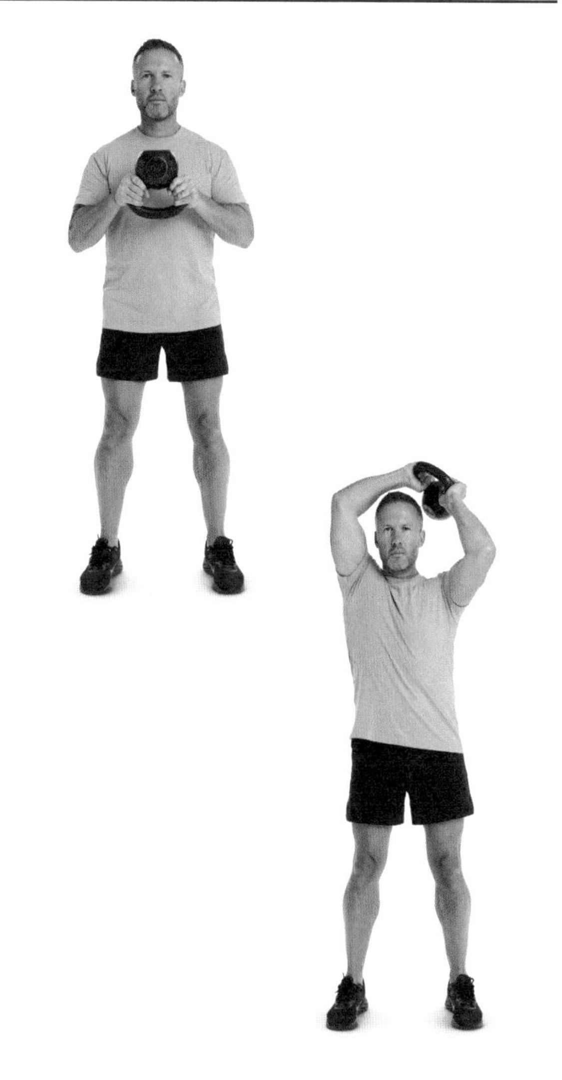

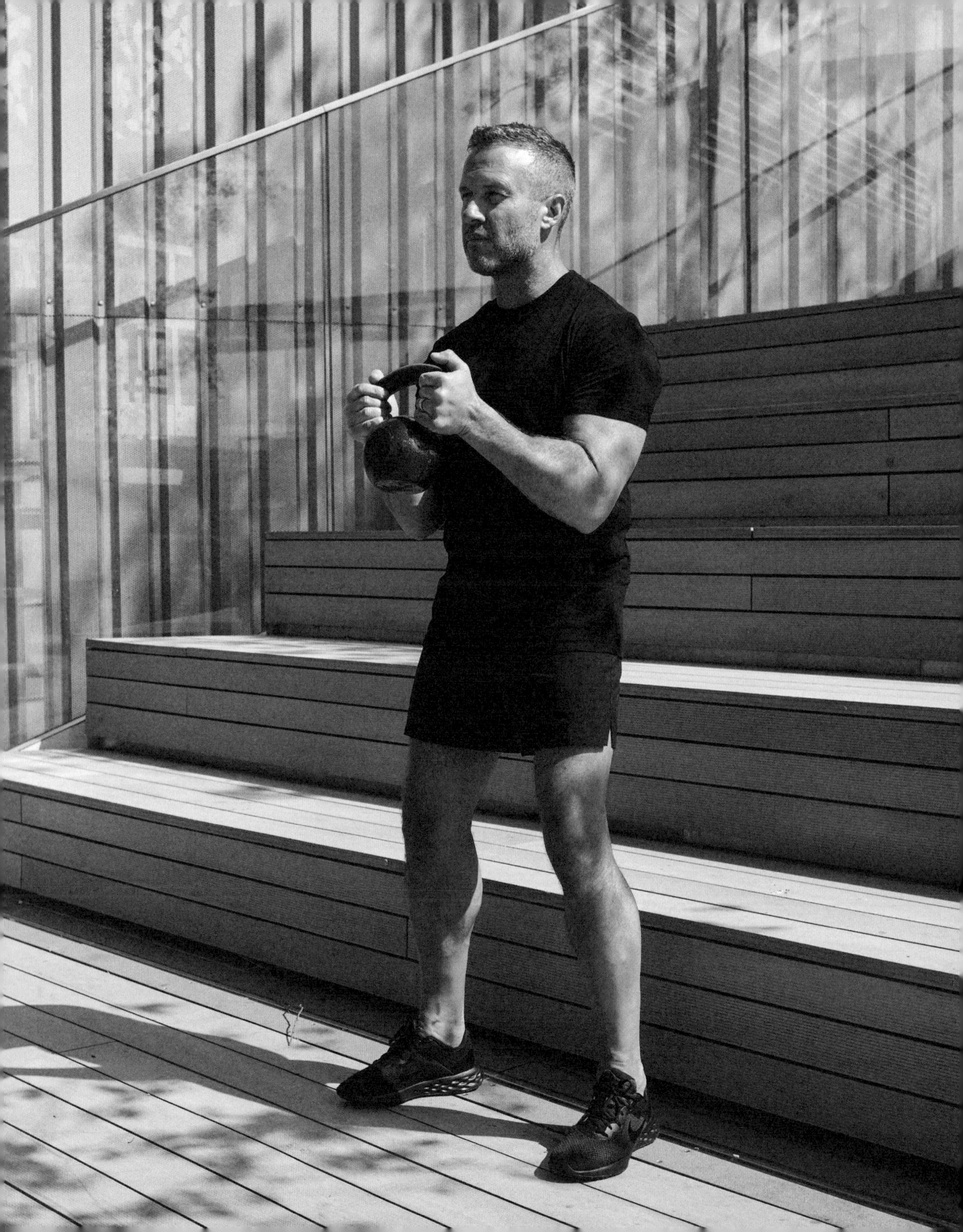

OVERHEAD PRESS

1 **START POSITION:** Stand with your feet shoulder-width apart, holding the kettlebell by the weighted ball at chest height.
2 Push the kettlebell overhead, then lower it back down to your chest.

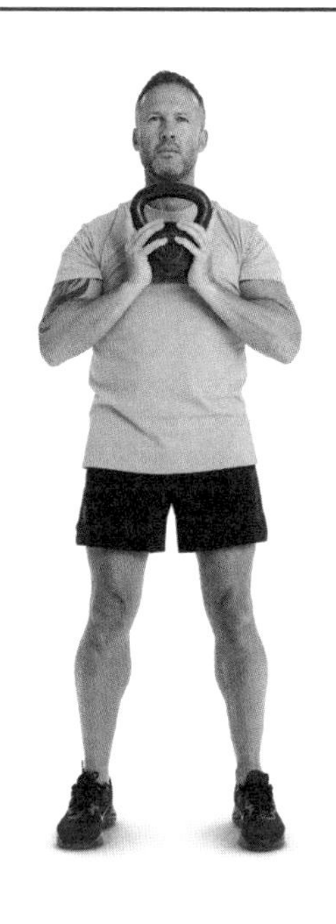

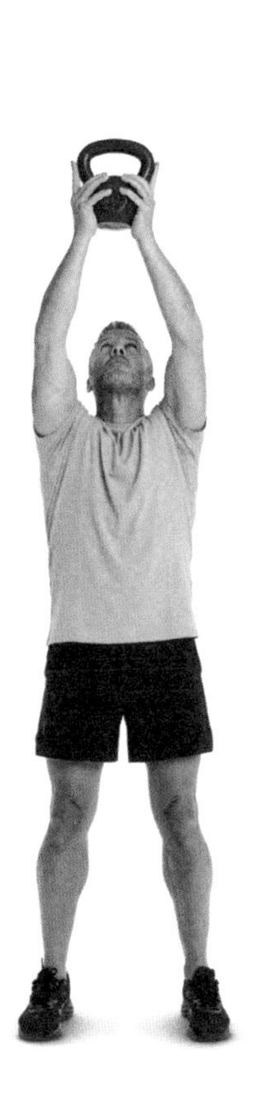

DEADLIFTS

1 **START POSITION:** Start with your feet shoulder-width apart with the kettlebell held down in front of you. Grip the kettlebell with two hands using an overhand grip.
2 Hinge at the hip and lower down, bending your knees until you are in a slight squat position, chest up, spine straight. Let the kettlebell touch the floor.
3 Drive up with your weight in your heels. Once the kettlebell reaches knee level, drive your hips forward and come to an upright position, squeezing your glutes.

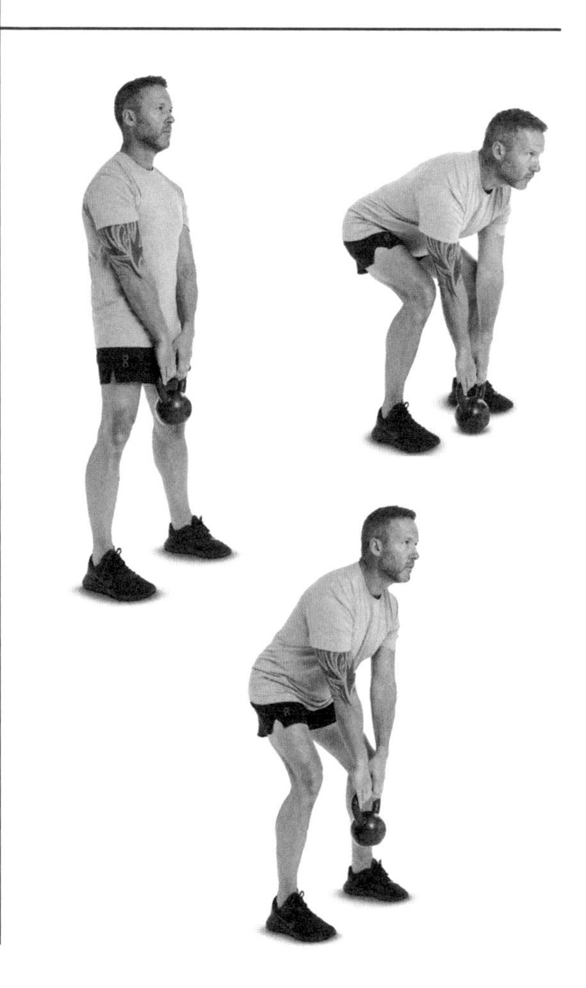

CHALLENGE 2

PUT YOUR BACK INTO IT

- **Not all workouts have to be fast and furious. When you slow your movements down and focus on spending more time under tension, you're working your body just as hard.**

- **Perform each exercise 12 times, resting for around 15–30 seconds between exercises.**

- **Repeat the sequence three times, resting as needed between each round.**

ALTERNATING GORILLA ROWS

1 **START POSITION:** Stand with your feet slightly wider than shoulder-width apart with the kettlebell placed centrally. Hinge at your hips and lean your body forwards until your chest is parallel to the ground. Keep your arms straight below your chest with palms facing each other. Brace your core, look down, and maintain a neutral spine position. Grip the kettlebell in your right hand, palm facing in. Pull your elbow up to the side keeping it tucked in.

2 Return the kettlebell to the start position on the floor and repeat on the opposite side.

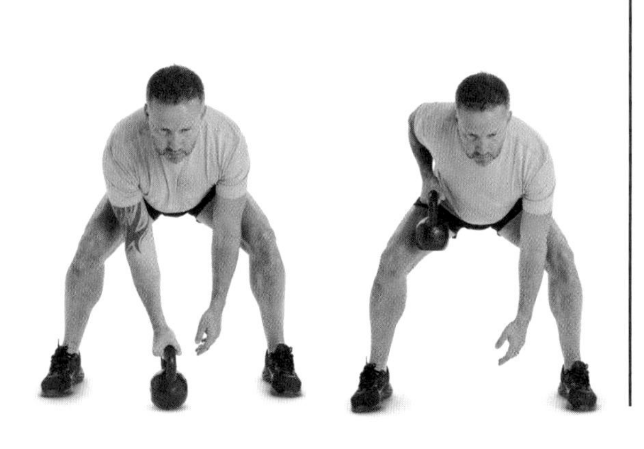

STRICT PRESS (LEFT & RIGHT)

1 **START POSITION:** Stand with your feet hip-width apart holding the kettlebell in your right hand. Rest the kettlebell on your right shoulder with your palm facing out.

2 Press the kettlebell straight up overhead, engaging the core. Return the kettlebell to shoulder height and repeat on the opposite side.

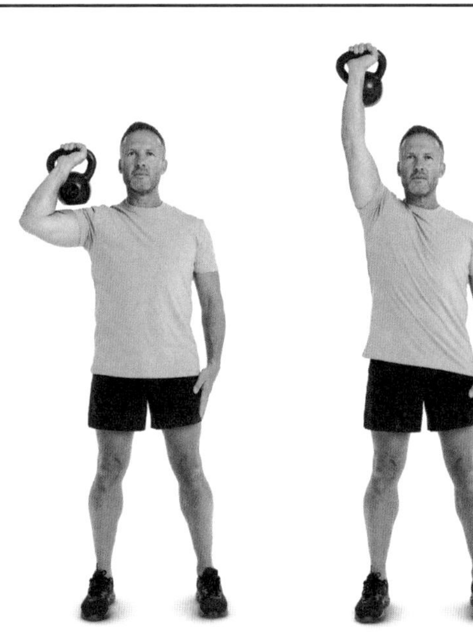

FIGURE-OF-EIGHTS

1 **START POSITION:** Stand with your feet slightly wider than shoulder-width apart. Pass the kettlebell from the right hand to the left hand, moving it in a circular path around the left leg.
2 Swing the kettlebell back between your legs, moving it behind the right leg, passing the kettlebell from the left hand to the right hand. Keep the kettlebell moving in a figure-of-eight path, passing it between hands.

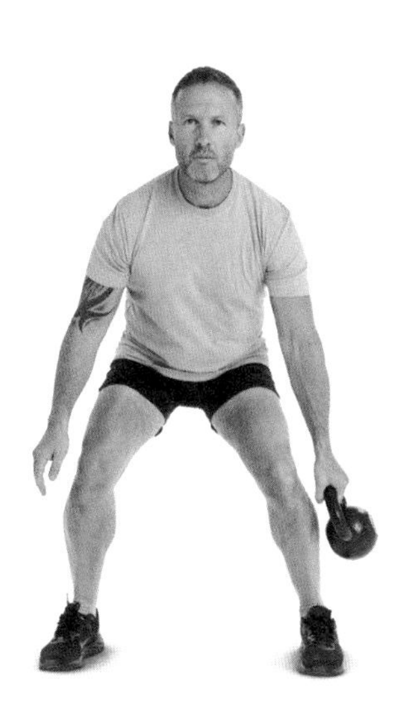

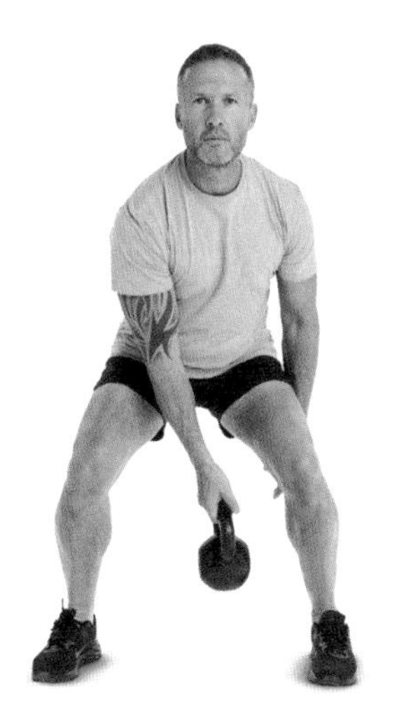

SUMO SQUATS

1 **START POSITION:** Start with your feet wider than shoulder-width apart with the kettlebell on the floor in front of you. Hinge at the hip and lower down, bending your knees until you are in a squat position with your chest up and your spine straight. Grip the kettlebell with two hands using an overhand grip. Drive up with your weight in your heels. Once the kettlebell reaches about knee level, drive your hips forwards as you come to an upright position, squeezing your glutes.
2 Slowly lower the kettlebell down by bending your knees until you are in a squat position with your chest up and your spine straight. Let the kettlebell touch the floor, pause in lowered position then repeat.

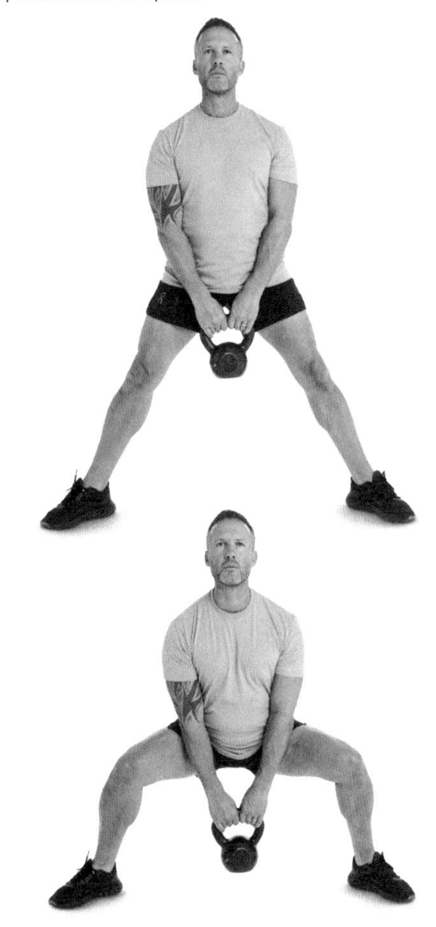

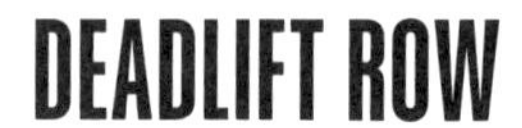

DEADLIFT ROW

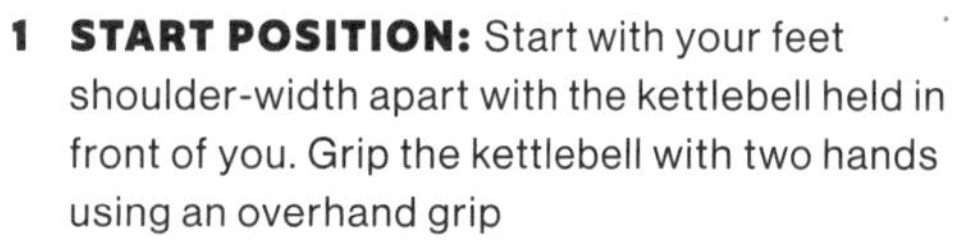

1 **START POSITION:** Start with your feet shoulder-width apart with the kettlebell held in front of you. Grip the kettlebell with two hands using an overhand grip
2 Hinge at the hip and lower down, bending your knees until you are in a squat position with your chest up and your spine straight.
3 Drive up with your weight through your heels. Once the kettlebell reaches about knee level, keeping the core engaged and back flat, pull the kettlebell up to your chest and then lower your arms back down.
4 Drive your hips forwards as you come back to an upright position, squeezing your glutes. Slowly lower the kettlebell down by bending your knees until you are in a squat position with your chest up and your spine straight. Let the kettlebell touch the floor, pause in lowered position, then repeat.

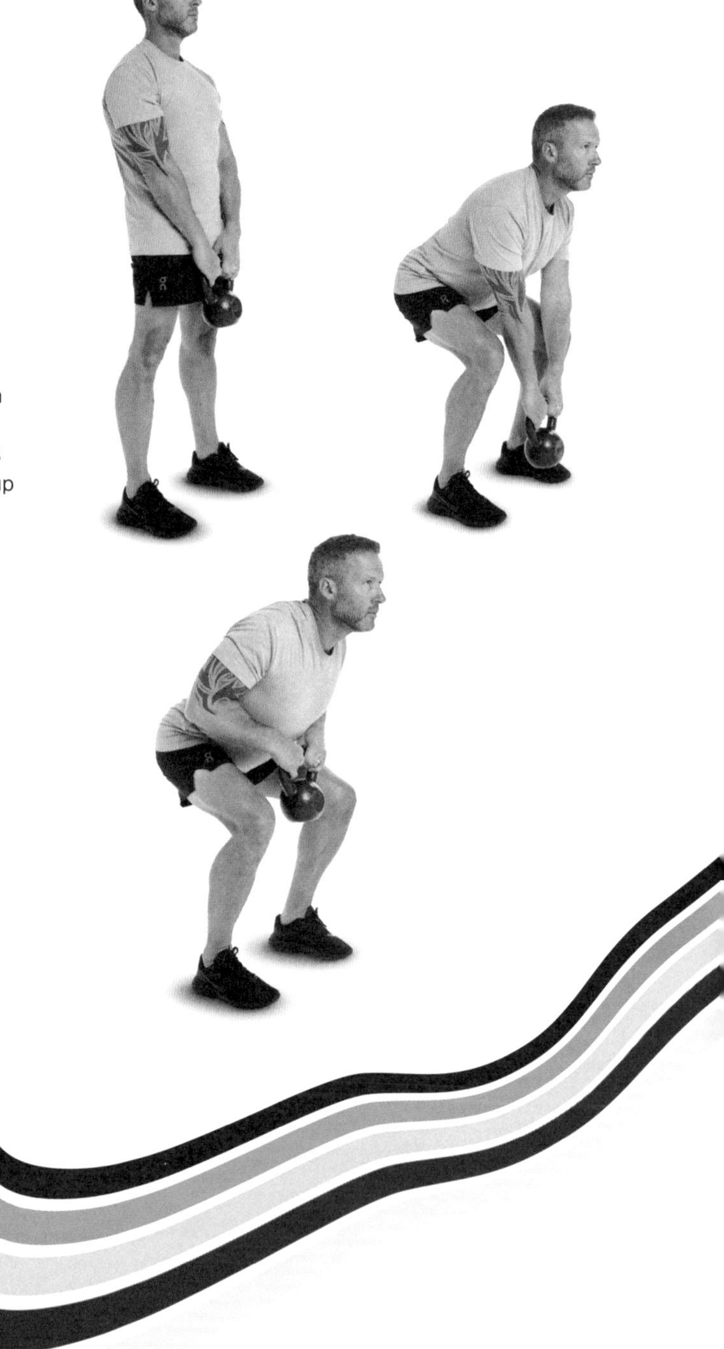

CHALLENGE 3

TWIST & SHOUT

- **This workout is designed to challenge the core and give the obliques some special attention. Keep your movements controlled.**
- **Do each exercise 10 times, resting as needed between each exercise.**
- **Aim for 15–30 seconds rest between each exercise then repeat the circuit 2–3 times, resting as needed between each circuit.**

HIGH KNEE TWIST

1. **START POSITION:** Start in a standing position with your feet hip-width apart, holding the kettlebell in front of your chest by the sides of its handle (horns). Tuck your elbows in.
2. Bring alternate knees up towards your chest as high as possible while moving the kettlebell to the opposite side.

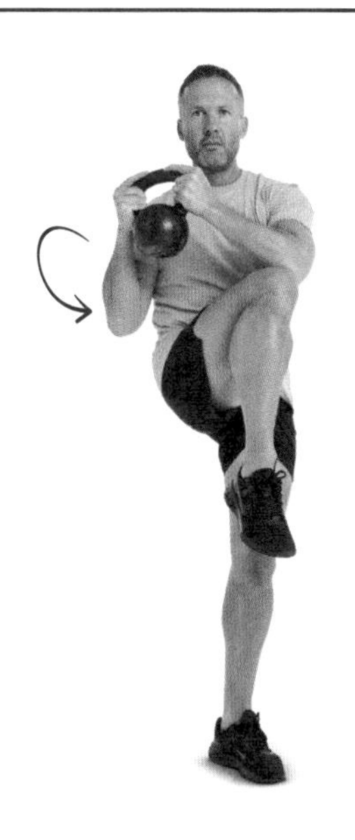

DEADBUG

1. **START POSITION:** Lie on your back with your arms at shoulder level raised towards the ceiling, holding the kettlebell with both hands. Bring your legs up into tabletop position, knees bent 90 degrees and in line with your hips.
2. Slowly extend your right leg out straight, while simultaneously lowering the kettlebell overhead. Keep both the arms and left leg extended just off the ground. Bring your arms and legs back to the starting position. Repeat on the opposite side.

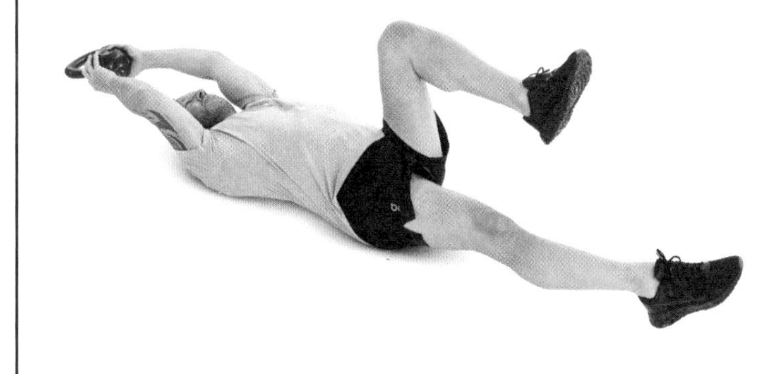

KNEELING WOODCHOPS (LEFT & RIGHT)

1 **START POSITION:** Start in a stable half kneeling position with your left knee at 90 degrees and your right knee supporting.
2 Bring the kettlebell to the hip where the knee is planted on the floor and rotate it up to the opposite side keeping your arms bent. Slowly return to the starting position with the kettlebell staying slightly away from the body. Repeat the whole exercise on the other side.

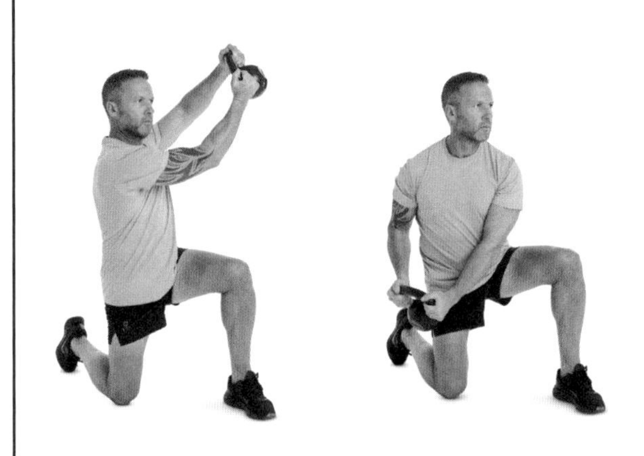

SIT UP PRESS

1 **START POSITION:** Lie down on your back, feet flat on the floor hip-width apart, knees bent. Find a comfortable and secure grip holding the kettlebell with both hands at your chest. Inhale and exhale and then lift your upper body, keeping your head and neck relaxed.
2 Push the kettlebell above your head, lower it back to the chest. Inhale and return to the starting position.

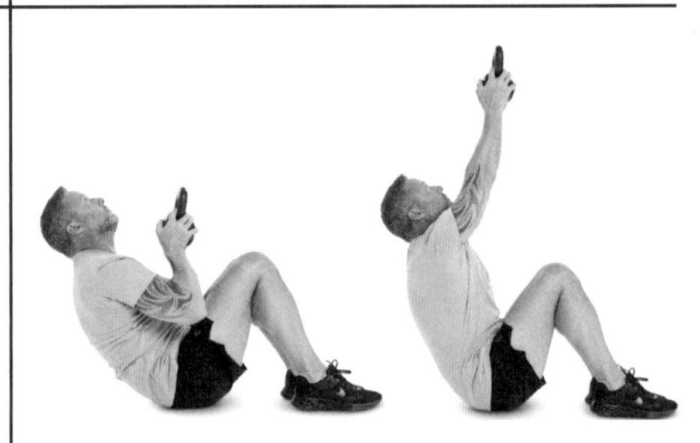

PULLOVERS WITH LEG RAISES

1 **START POSITION:** Lie on your back, feet flat on the floor hip-width apart, knees bent. Find a comfortable and secure grip holding the kettlebell with both hands raised up above your chest.
2 Extend your legs and lower the weight behind your head until it is just above the ground. Hold the tension for a moment.
3 Keeping your lower back pressed into the floor, bring the weight back up over your chest and raise your legs. Repeat.

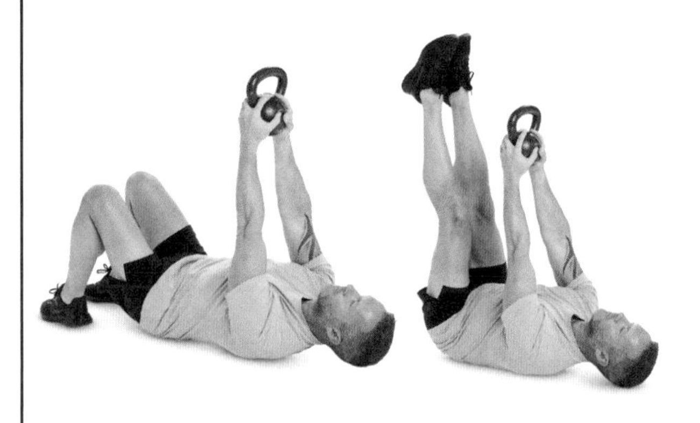

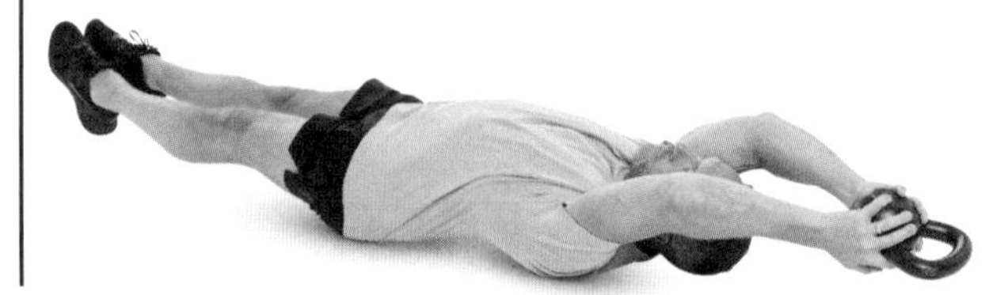

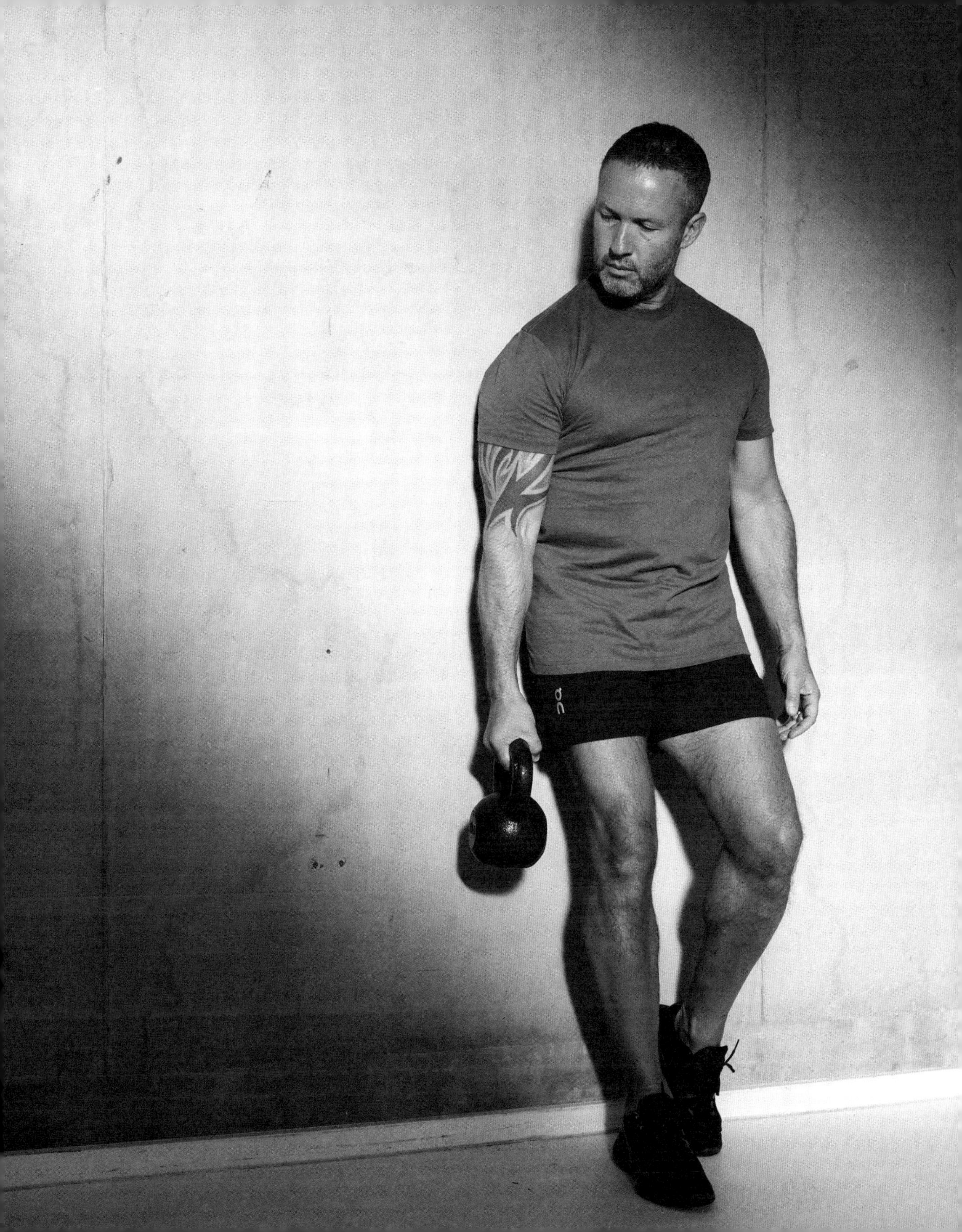

CHALLENGE 4

KING OF THE SWINGERS

- Hit the upper and lower body with this challenge, getting your heart rate up by swinging the kettlebell and getting some power through the legs.
- Perform the exercises for 40 seconds, then rest for 20 seconds.
- Complete as many rounds as possible in your time slot.

KETTLEBELL SWINGS

1. **START POSITION:** Stand with your back straight and feet shoulder-width apart holding the kettlebell with both hands, arms extended.
2. Engage your core, bend your knees as you straighten your legs, push from the heels and through the hips, swinging the kettlebell to chest height. As you swing the kettlebell down between your legs, return to the half-squat position.

SUMO SQUATS

1. **START POSITION:** Start with your feet wider than shoulder-width apart with the kettlebell on the floor in front of you. Hinge at the hip and lower down, bending your knees until you are in a squat position with your chest up and your spine straight. Grip the kettlebell with two hands using an overhand grip. Drive up with your weight in your heels. Once the kettlebell reaches about knee level, drive your hips forwards as you come to an upright position, squeezing your glutes.
2. Slowly lower the kettlebell down by bending your knees until you are in a squat position with your chest up and your spine straight. Let the kettlebell touch the floor, pause in lowered position then repeat.

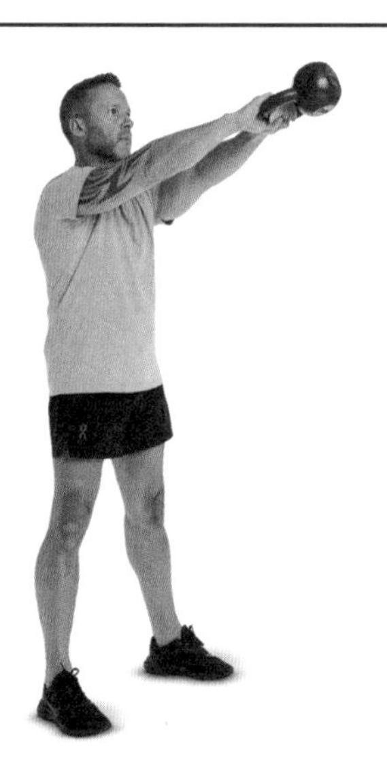

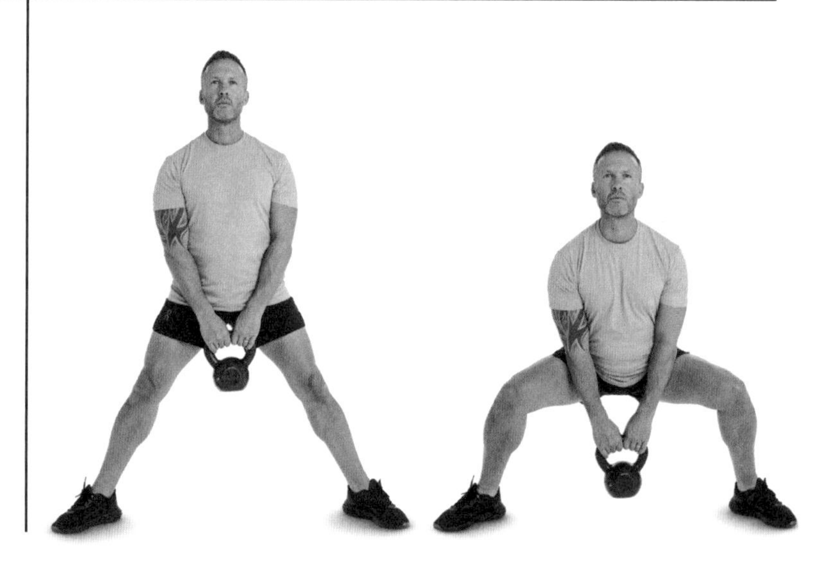

SINGLE ARM SWINGS (RIGHT AND LEFT)

1. **START POSITION:** Stand with your back straight and your feet shoulder-width apart, holding the kettlebell in your right hand with your arm extended.
2. Engaging your core, bend your knees as you straighten your legs, push from the heels and explode through the hips and swing the kettlebell to chest height. As you swing the kettlebell down between your legs, return to the half-squat position and repeat on the opposite side.

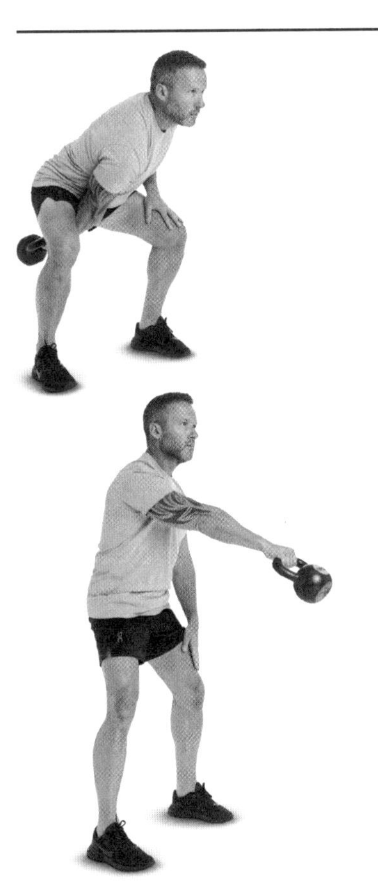

HAND-TO-HAND SWINGS

1. **START POSITION:** Stand with your back straight and feet shoulder-width apart, holding the kettlebell in one hand, arm extended. Engage your core, bend your knees as you straighten your leg push from the heels and explode through the hips, swinging the kettlebell to chest height. Exchange grip from one hand to the other.
2. As you swing the kettlebell down between your legs, return to the half-squat position and repeat, alternating between each hand.

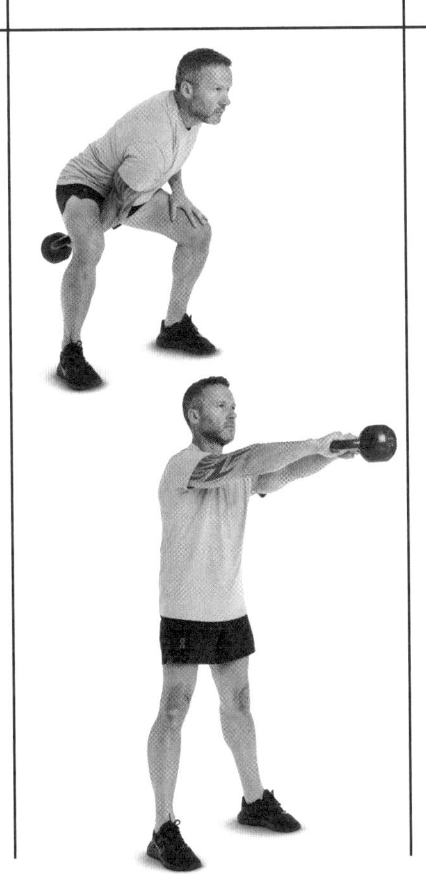

GOBLET SQUATS TO OVERHEAD PRESS

1. **START POSITION:** Stand with your feet shoulder-width apart. Hold the kettlebell in front of your chest by the sides of its handle (horns). Tuck your elbows in.
2. Keeping your back straight and your core engaged, push your hips back and squat down, as if you were sitting down into a chair.
3. Drive your weight through your heels back to a standing position and push the kettlebell overhead, then lower it back the chest. Repeat.

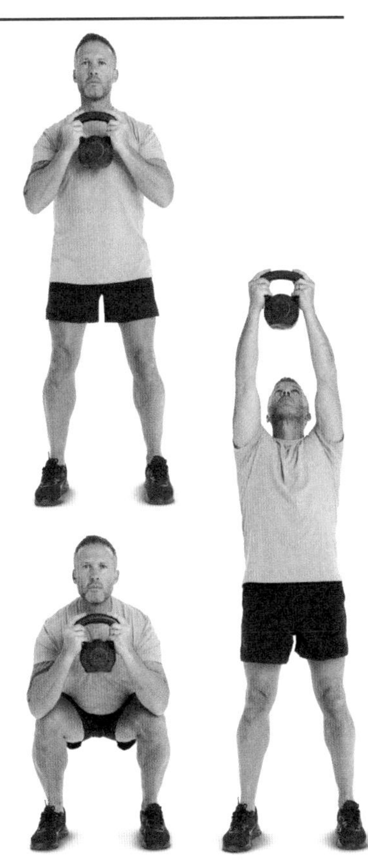

CHALLENGE 5

TWENTY TEN TIME

- **TABATA TIME** – Tabata is a high-intensity interval training style that squeezes Herculean effort into a short amount of time.
- 20 seconds maximum effort followed by 10 seconds rest.
- Perform the first two exercises for 4 minutes. Rest for a full minute before moving on to the next pair of exercises.

MOUNTAIN CLIMBERS

1 **START POSITION:** Start in a high plank position.
2 Bring your left knee towards your chest, then switch legs and bring your right knee towards your chest. Keep switching legs as though you're running in place.

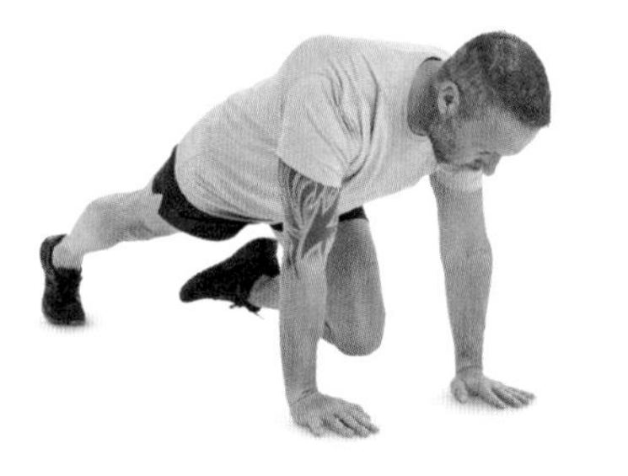

ALTERNATING HAMMER CURLS

1 **START POSITION:** Start in a standing position with your feet hip-width apart. With your arms down by your sides, turn your hands palms inwards, holding the kettlebell in a neutral grip. Pull your shoulders down and back and brace your core.
2 Bend your elbows and curl the weight up until your forearm is just above parallel to the floor. Keep your wrists straight. Lower the kettlebell, swap to the other hand and repeat.

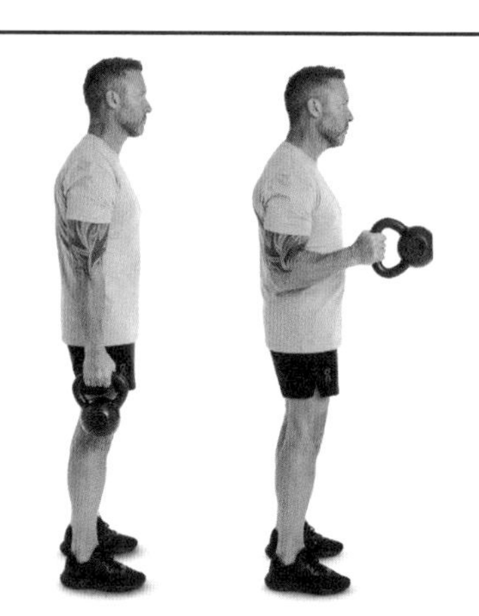

HIGH KNEES

1 **START POSITION:** Start in a standing position with your feet hip-width apart. Run in place, bringing your knees up towards your chest as high as possible while pumping your arms.
2 Keep your chest lifted and your core engaged, using the ball of each foot to launch into the next step.

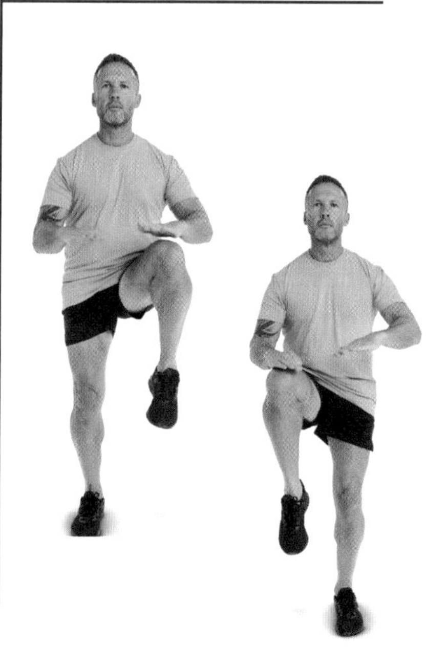

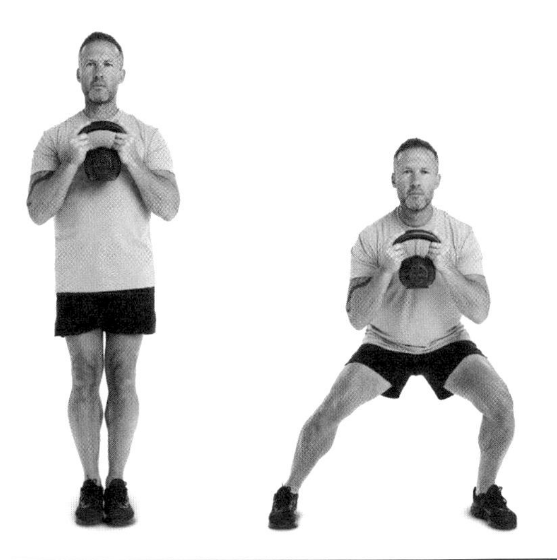

BOB AND WEAVE

1 **START POSITION:** Stand with your feet together and the kettlebell held in both hands by the horns at chest height.
2 Take a wide step to the left coming to a squat position, bring the legs back together and repeat on the right, keeping the kettlebell held in front of your chest.

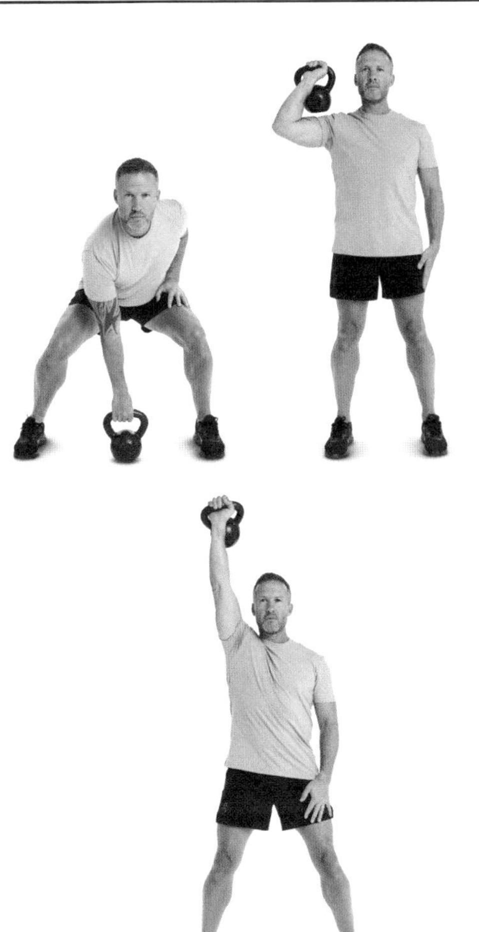

ALTERNATING CLEAN AND PRESS

1 **START POSITION:** Stand with your feet hip-width apart with the kettlebell between your feet. Bend down and grip the kettlebell at the end of the handle with your right hand. Drive through your glutes to stand up and bring the kettlebell up so it's resting on the outside of your forearm. Slightly bend your knees, keeping your chest upright.
2 Push the kettlebell up overhead as you drive up through your glutes to standing.
3 Return the kettlebell to the start position on the floor and repeat on the opposite side.

BURPEES

1. **START POSITION:** Stand feet shoulder-width apart.
2. Bend your knees and reach forwards to place your hands on the floor.
3. Kick both legs straight out behind you into a high plank position.
4. Hop your legs back under your body.
5. Jump straight up into the air, reaching your arms overhead. Land with your knees slightly bent.

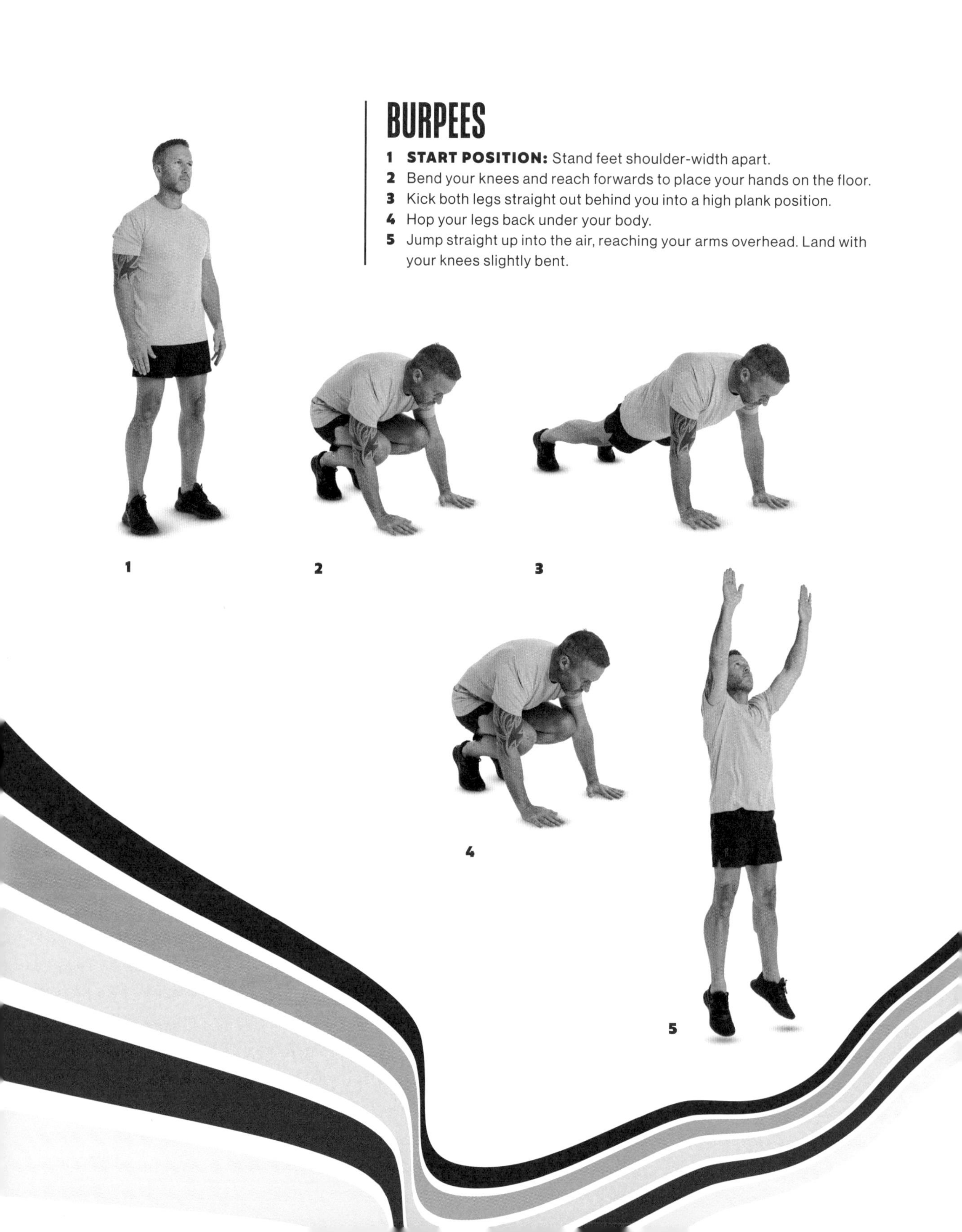

CHALLENGE 6

CORE CONNECTION

- From injury prevention to activities for daily living, a strong core is essential. We're going to hit the floor to work from top-to-toe with a focus on strengthening that centre connection.
- Perform each exercise 20 times, resting as needed between exercises.
- Rinse and repeat for a total of 2 rounds, 3 rounds for an extra burn.

PLANK TAPS

1. **START POSITION:** Start in a high plank position with your feet slightly wider than hip-width apart and a kettlebell placed directly in front of you so you can just reach it.
2. Tap each hand to the kettlebell while engaging your core to keep the hips as still as possible.

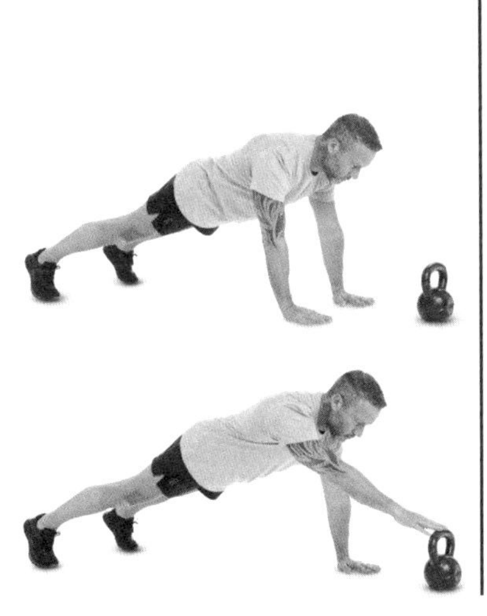

FLUTTER KICKS

1. **START POSITION:** Lie on your back with your legs straight out in front. Hold the kettlebell with both hands directly above your chest, with straight arms.
2. Lift your head and shoulders, engage the core to keep your back pushed into the floor. Raise your feet and kick up and down in a swimming motion.

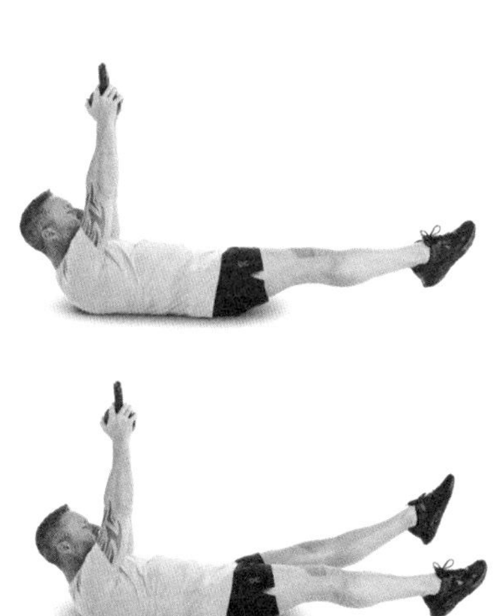

INCLINE PRESS

1. **START POSITION:** Start in a seated position with knees bent in front of you, holding the kettlebell with both hands. Lean back slightly so your body and legs form a V shape, engaging your core.
2. Extend your arms so the kettlebell is above your chest. Lower with control to touch the chest and repeat.

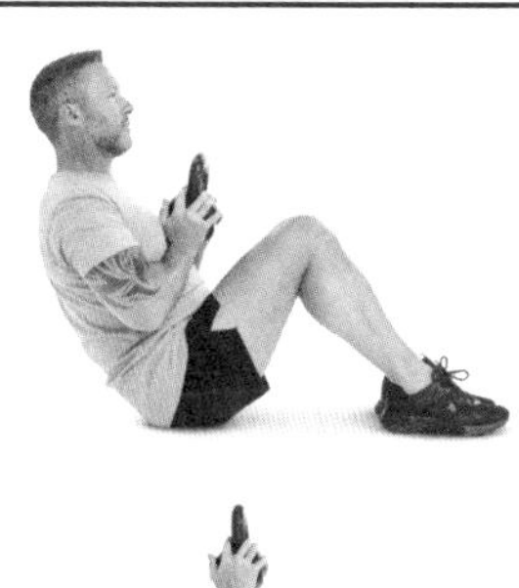

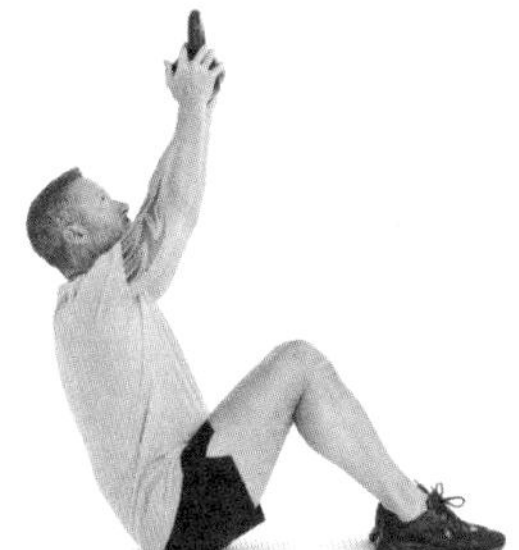

RUSSIAN TWISTS

1 **START POSITION:** Sit on the floor with your legs out in front of you with your knees bent, heels down. Lean back slightly so your body and legs form a V shape, engaging your core.
2 Twist your torso from side to side, keeping your core strong and your knees bent, don't let them move from side to side.

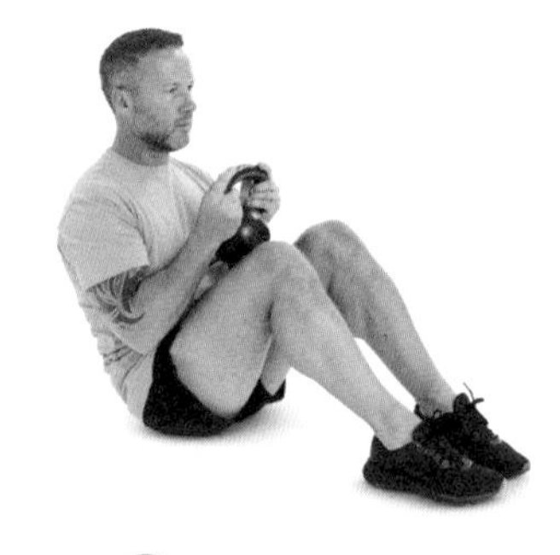

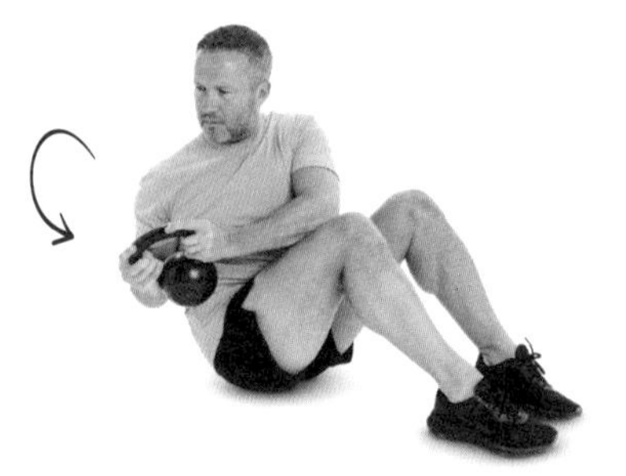

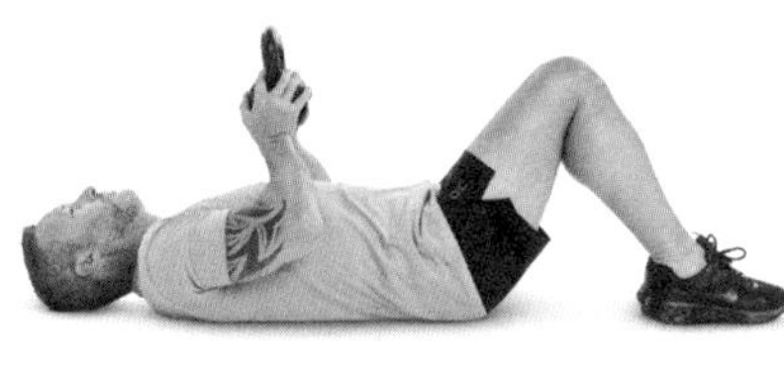

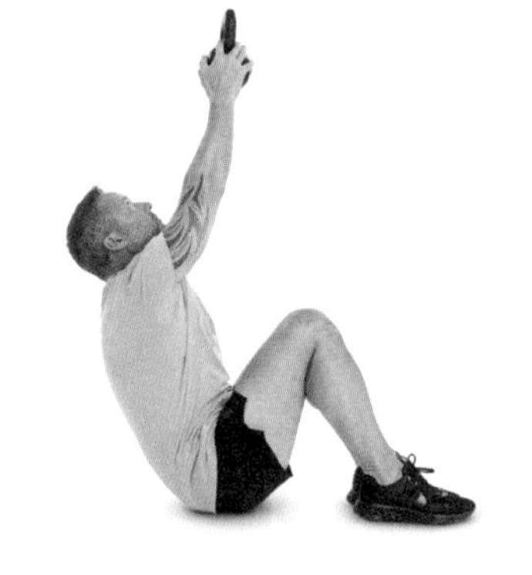

SIT UP PRESS

1 **START POSITION:** Lie down on your back, feet flat on the floor hip-width apart, knees bent. Find a comfortable and secure grip holding the kettlebell with both hands at your chest. Inhale and exhale and then lift your upper body, keeping your head and neck relaxed.
2 Push the kettlebell above your head, lower back the chest. Inhale and return to the starting position.

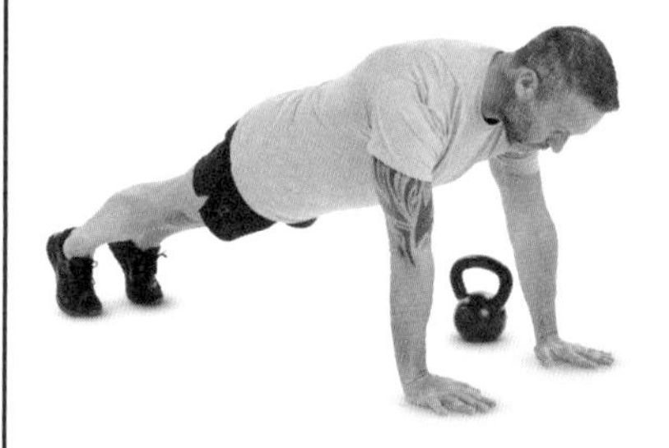

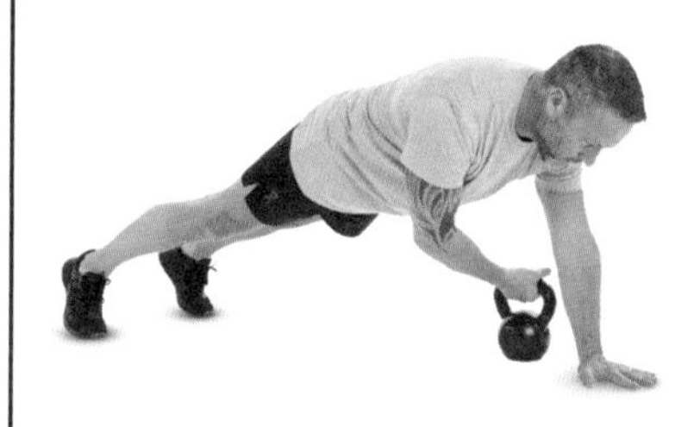

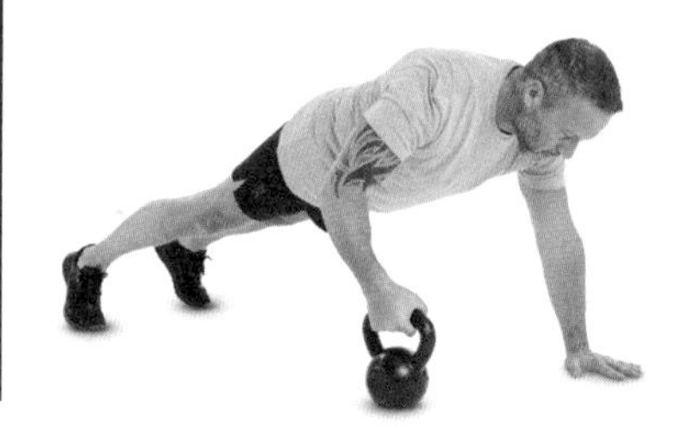

PLANK DRAGS

1 **START POSITION:** Start in a high plank position with your feet slightly wider than hip-width apart and the kettlebell placed slightly outside the elbow.
2 Reach through with the opposing arm and drag the kettlebell through to the other side of your body.
3 Release the kettlebell, place your hand on the floor and then drag the kettlebell back to the other side of your body with the other hand.

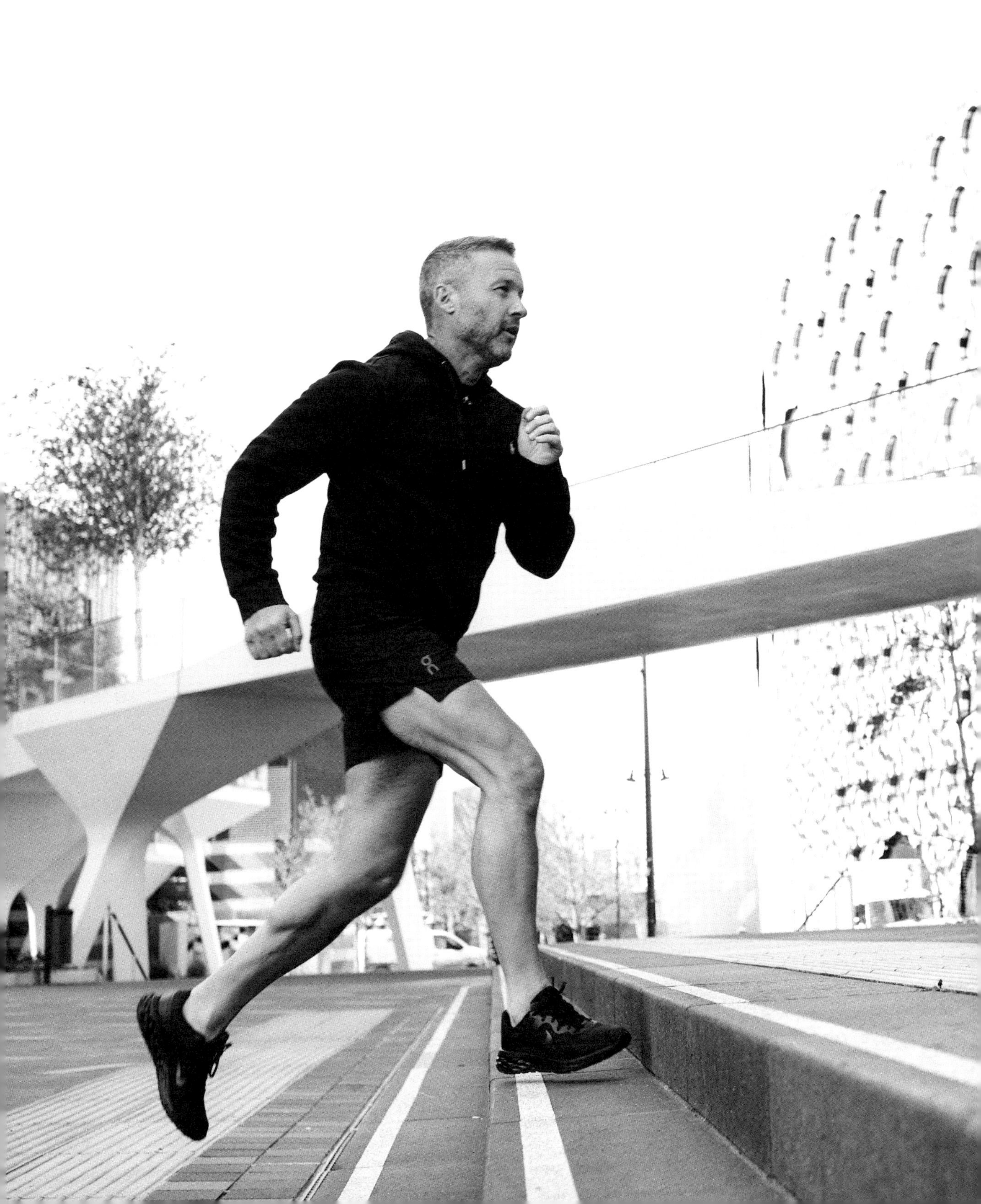

CHALLENGE 7

EAT, SLEEP, REP, REPEAT

- When you feel the need to kick-start those feel-good endorphins then try this high-energy blast to work your body from head to toe.
- Perform each exercise 10 times and complete as many rounds as you can in 20 minutes.

LATERAL SWINGS (LEFT & RIGHT)

1. **START POSITION:** Stand with a wide stance, feet wider than shoulder-width apart. Hold the kettlebell in your left hand with a straight arm. Slightly swing it to the left, then drive the kettlebell across to the right.
2. As the kettlebell goes up to shoulder height, straighten your legs and squeeze your glutes.
3. Bring the kettlebell down across your body to just below and outside the left knee, bending your knees as you do so.
4. Repeat the whole exercise on the other side.

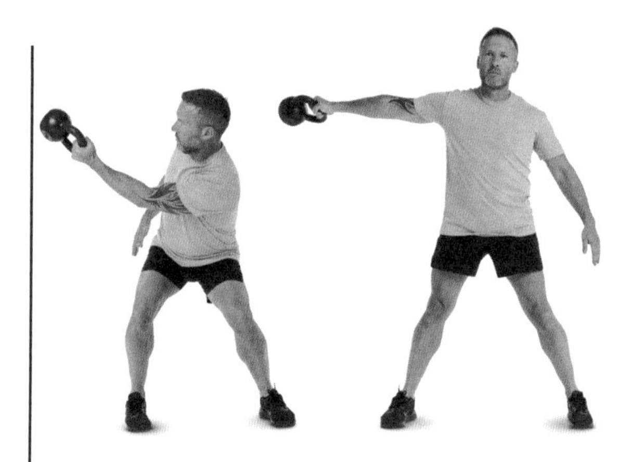

THRUSTERS

1. **START POSITION:** Stand with your feet slightly wider than hip-width apart, holding the kettlebell in front of you at chest height.
2. Push your bottom back and bend your knees until your thighs are parallel to the ground, keeping your back straight and your chest up.
3. Push through your heels back to standing, raising the kettlebell overhead.
4. Return the kettlebell to chest height and repeat.

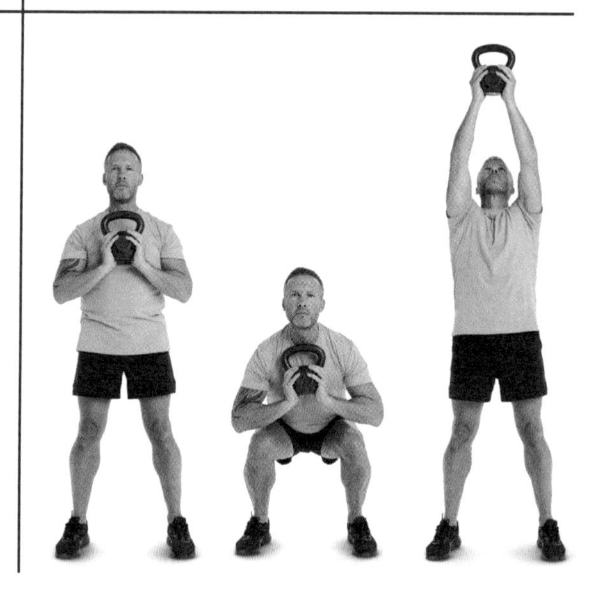

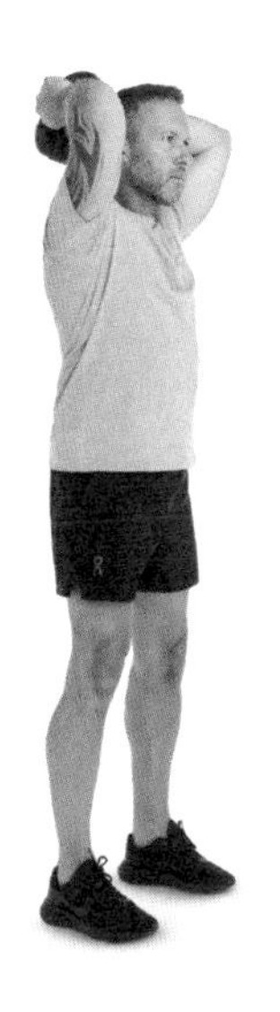

OVERHEAD TRICEP EXTENSIONS

1 **START POSITION:** Stand with your feet shoulder-width apart holding the kettlebell reverse grip by the horns above the head.
2 Lower the kettlebell with control behind your head, keeping your elbows facing forwards.
3 Push the kettlebell back overhead to the starting position and repeat.

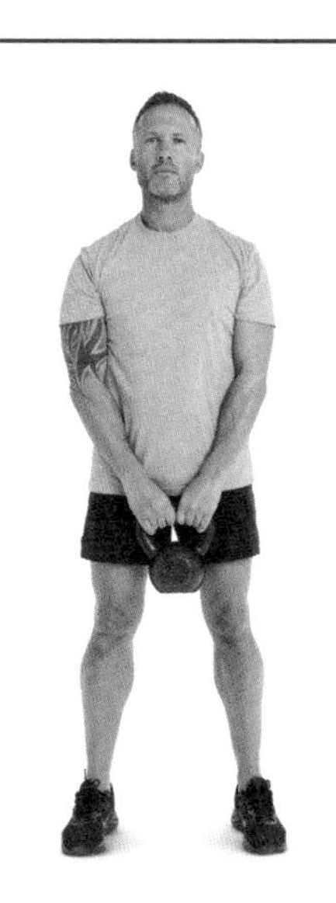

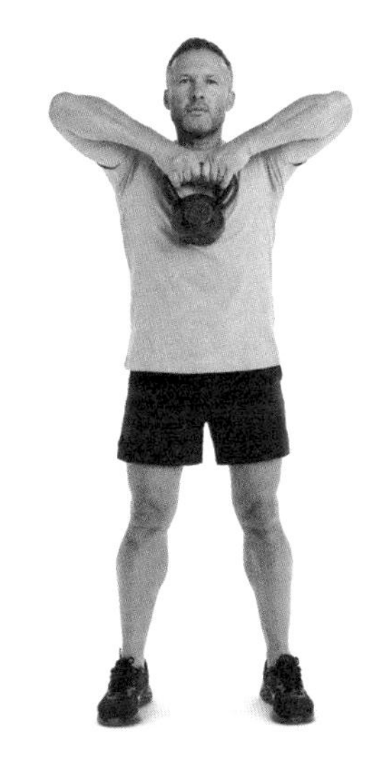

TRAP ROWS

1 **START POSITION:** Stand with feet shoulder-width apart, holding the kettlebell by the handle with both hands, palms facing in and arms extended.
2 Pull the kettlebell towards your chin, keeping the elbows wide. When the kettlebell is at about chest height, pause, then slowly lower your arms back down until they reach full extension. Repeat.

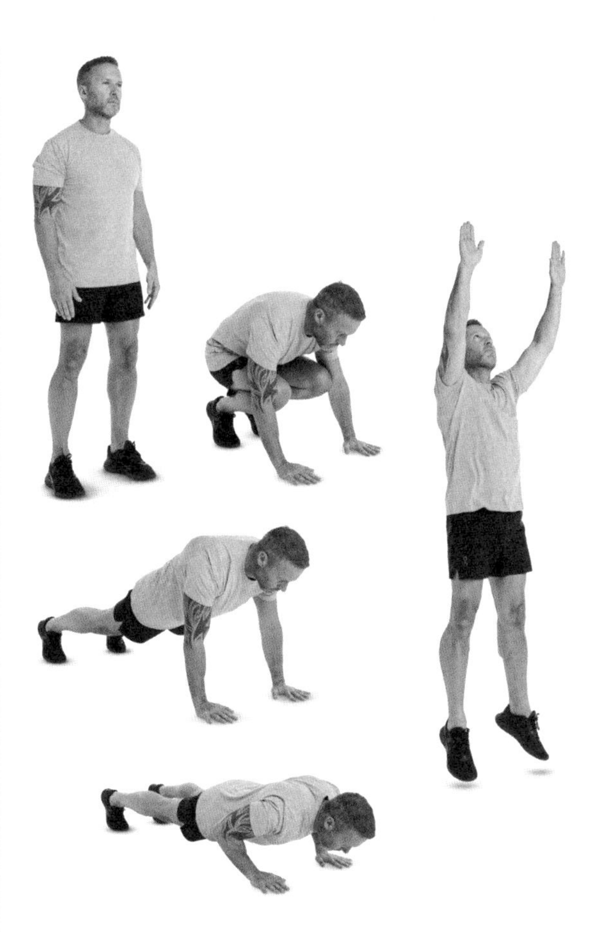

PUSH-UP BURPEES

1 **START POSITION:** Stand with your feet shoulder-width apart.
2 Bend your knees and reach forwards to place your hands on the floor.
3 Kick both legs straight out behind you into a high plank position.
4 Lower to a plank, holding your body parallel to the floor.
5 Hop your legs back under your body and jump straight up into the air, reaching your arms overhead. Land with your knees slightly bent.

CHALLENGE 8

IT'S ALL GONE SIDEWAYS

- These exercises are all about strong and controlled movements. Slow everything down and take your time to feel the mind to muscle connection.
- Perform each exercise 10 times then repeat the sequence 3 times, resting as needed.
- Don't rush as you move between exercises.

ALTERNATING CLEAN AND PRESS

1. **START POSITION:** Stand with your feet hip-width apart with the kettlebell between your feet, turned sideways. Bend down and grip the kettlebell at the end of the handle with your right hand.
2. Drive through your glutes to stand up and bring the kettlebell up so it's resting on the outside of your right forearm. Slightly bend your knees, keeping your chest upright.
3. Push the kettlebell up overhead as you drive up through your glutes to standing. Return the kettlebell to the starting position on the floor and repeat on the opposite side.

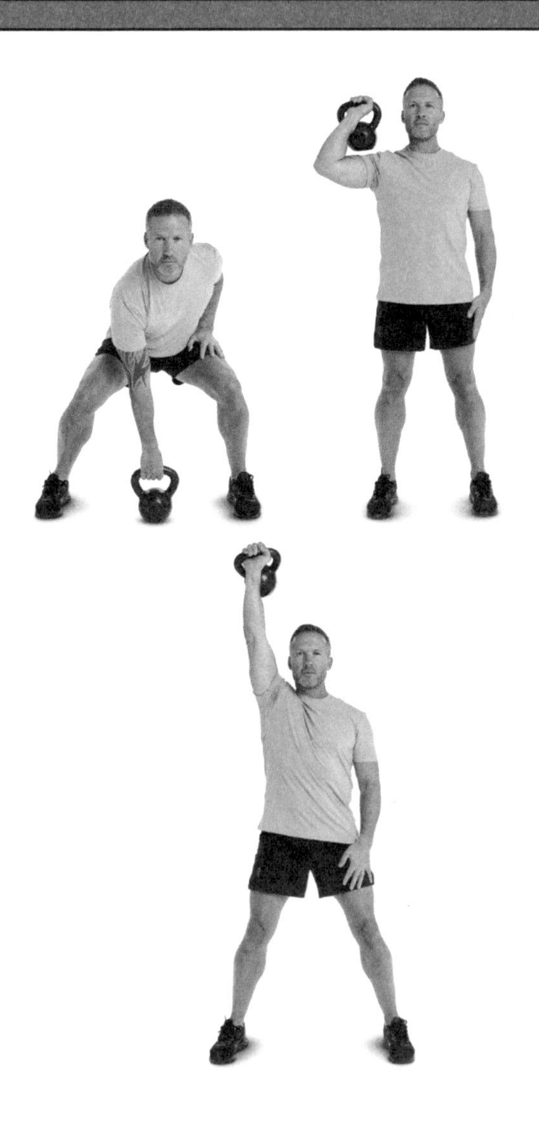

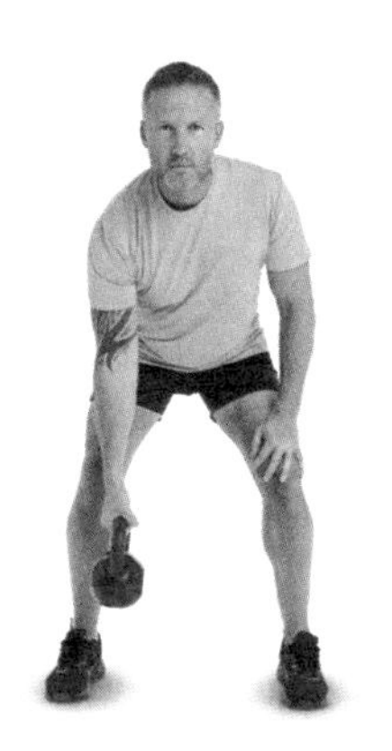
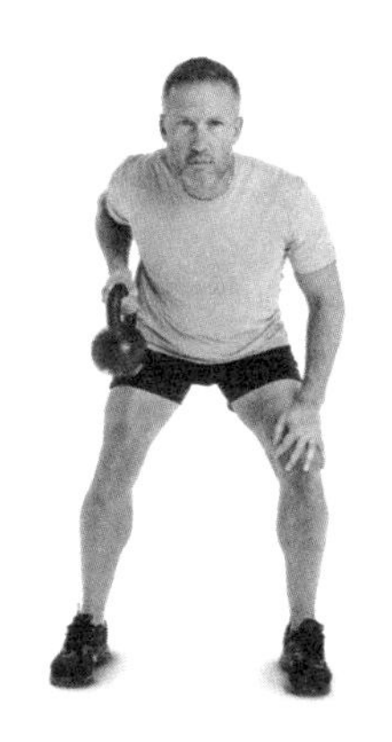

BENT OVER ROWS (LEFT & RIGHT)

1 **START POSITION:** Stand with your feet hip-width width apart and hold the kettlebell in a neutral grip in your right hand, palm facing in. Hinge your torso forwards to 45-degrees with right arm straight and a slight bend in your knees.
2 Pull the kettlebell up to your chest and then lower your arm back down and repeat.
3 Swap hands and repeat on the opposite side.

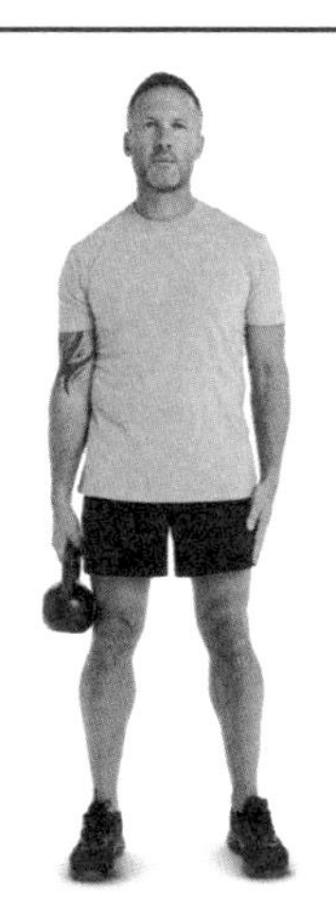
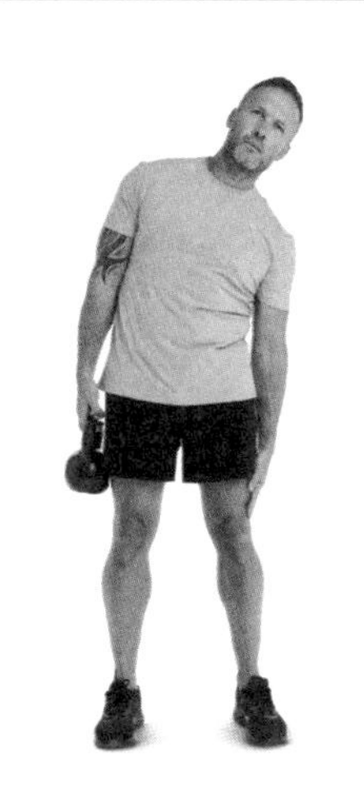

SIDE BENDS (LEFT & RIGHT)

1 **START POSITION:** Stand with your legs hip- to shoulder-width apart, holding the kettlebell in your right hand, palm facing in.
2 Bend as far to the left side as you can while maintaining a straight back and keeping your core active. Return to the start position and repeat.
3 Swap hands and repeat on the opposite side.

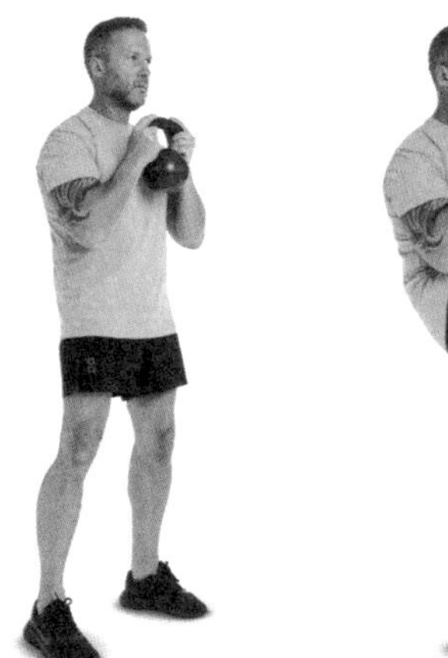
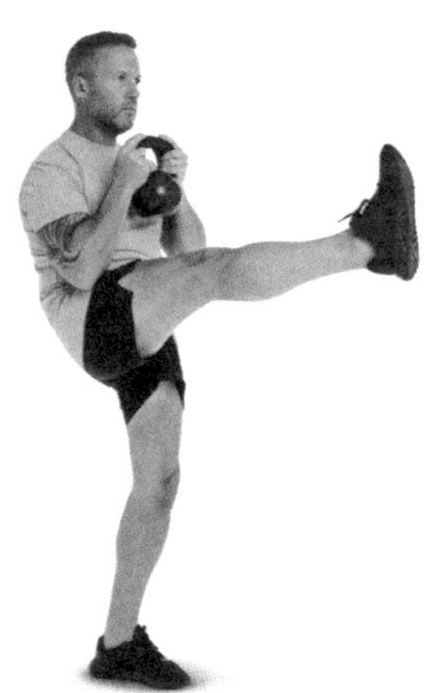

KETTLEBELL KICKS

1 **START POSITION:** Start in a standing position with your feet hip-width apart, holding the kettlebell in front of your chest by the sides of its handle. Tuck your elbows in. Slightly bend your knees, keeping your chest upright.
2 Kick your right leg straight out in front. Squeeze your glutes and keep your core tight. Lower your right leg and repeat with the left leg, keeping the kettlebell at chest height and engaging the core.

CHALLENGE 9

GROUND ZERO

- **Don't think that because you're hitting the floor for this circuit it will be easier than standing! This is great teamed up with one of our fast and furious circuits for a super set!**
- **Perform 5 reps of each exercise with minimal rest between.**
- **Complete 2–4 rounds.**

ONE ARM FLOOR PRESS (LEFT & RIGHT)

1 **START POSITION:** Lie on your back with your knees bent and feet flat on the floor. Holding the kettlebell in your right hand with your elbow touching the floor.
2 Press your arm to full extension and then return to the starting position.
3 Swap hands and repeat on the opposite side.

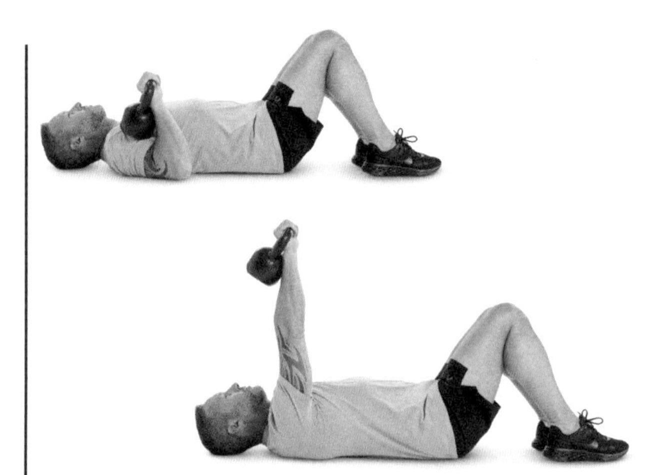

PULL OVERS

1 **START POSITION:** Lie on your back, feet flat on the floor hip-width apart, knees bent. Find a comfortable and secure grip holding the kettlebell with both hands at your chest. Lower the weight behind your head until it is just above the ground and hold the tension for a moment.
2 Keeping the lower back pressed into the floor, bring the weight back up. Repeat.

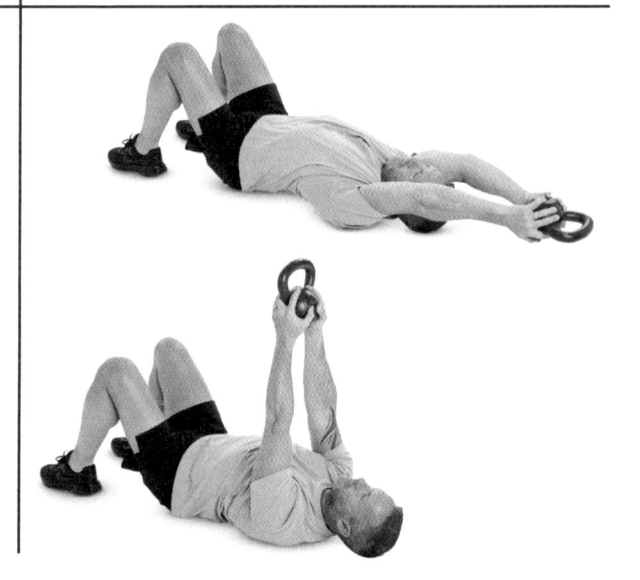

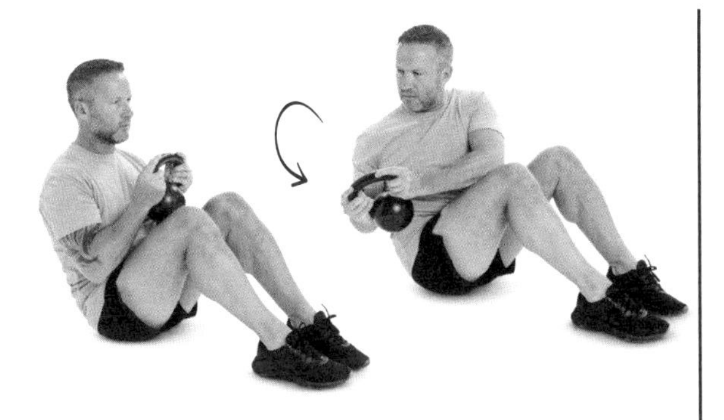

RUSSIAN TWISTS

1. **START POSITION:** Sit on the floor with your legs out in front of you with your knees bent, heels down. Lean back slightly so your body and legs form a V shape, engaging your core.
2. Twist your torso from side to side, keeping your core strong and your knees bent, don't let them move from side to side.

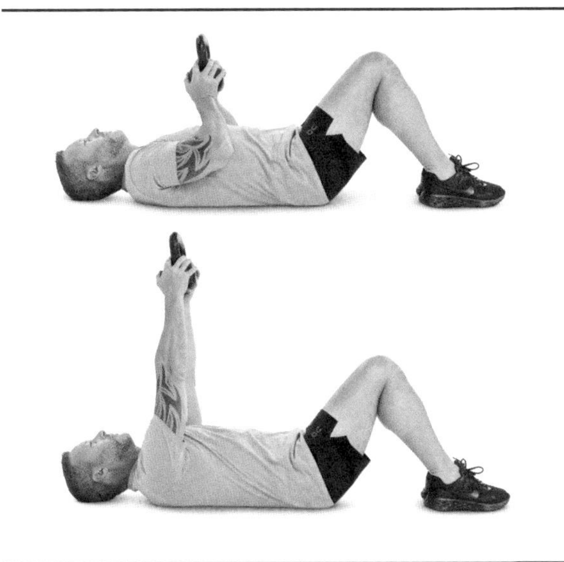

FLOOR PRESS

1. **START POSITION:** Lie on your back with your knees bent and feet flat on the floor. Hold the kettlebell in both hands above your chest.
2. Push the kettlebell up until your arms are fully extended, then return to the starting position. Repeat.

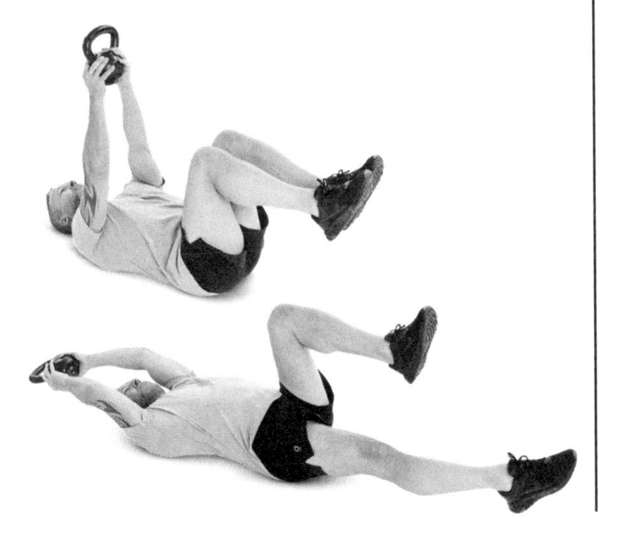

DEADBUGS

1. **START POSITION:** Lie on your back with your arms at shoulder level raised towards the ceiling, holding the kettlebell in both hands. Bring your legs up into tabletop position, knees bent 90 degrees in line with your hips.
2. Slowly extend your right leg out straight and bring the kettlebell overhead. Keep your right leg and arms just off the ground. Bring your arms and leg back to the starting position. Repeat on the opposite side.

CHALLENGE 10

PERFECTLY BALANCED

- **These movements work on balance and stability while sculpting and toning.**
- **Perform each kettlebell exercise 12 times.**
- **Hit those High Knees and Fast Feet for 1 minute each in between alternating the left and right versions of kneeling rotations and bottom up press. Two rounds is great, three is AWESOME.**

KNEELING ROTATIONS (LEFT & RIGHT)

1 **START POSITION:** Start in a stable half-kneeling position with your left knee at 90 degrees and right knee supporting. Rest the kettlebell on your right shoulder, palm facing out.
2 Rotate to the left, return to centre and press the kettlebell straight up overhead, engaging the core. Return the kettlebell to shoulder height and repeat.
3 Change to the opposite knee and swap hands to repeat on other side.

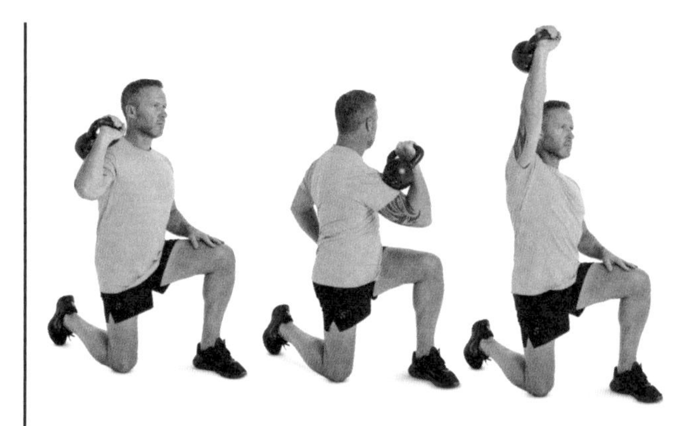

HIGH KNEES

1 **START POSITION:** Start in a standing position with your feet hip-width apart. Run in place, bringing your knees up towards your chest as high as possible while pumping your arms.
2 Keep your chest lifted and your core engaged, using the ball of your foot to launch into the next step.

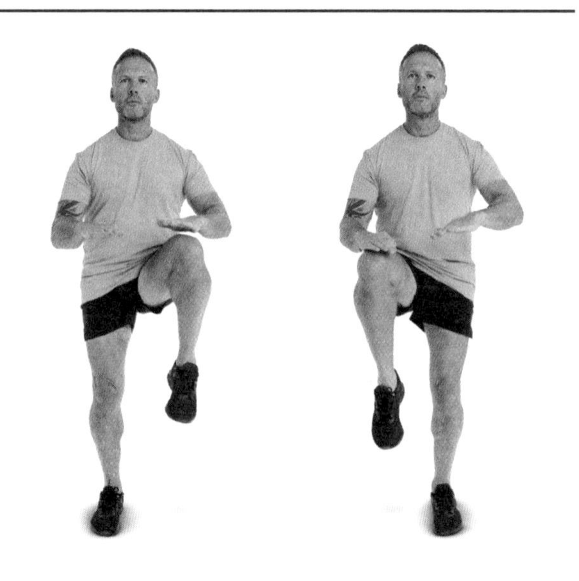

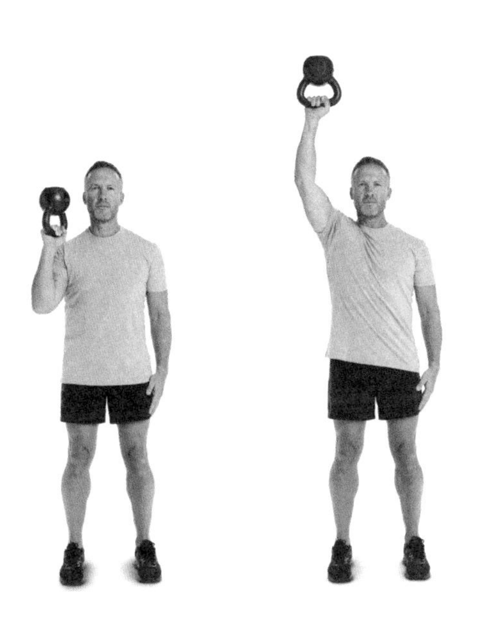

BOTTOM UP PRESS (LEFT & RIGHT)

1. **START POSITION:** Stand with your feet shoulder-width apart, holding the kettlebell in your right hand. Bring it to shoulder height, gripping it by the handle in one hand with the ball of the kettlebell pointing up. Engage your core and tighten your glutes and thighs.
2. Keeping your wrist in line with your elbow, press the kettlebell overhead with control, pause at the top with your arm extended, arm close to your ear. Bend your elbow and lower the kettlebell back to the starting position with control.
3. Swap hands and repeat on the opposite side.

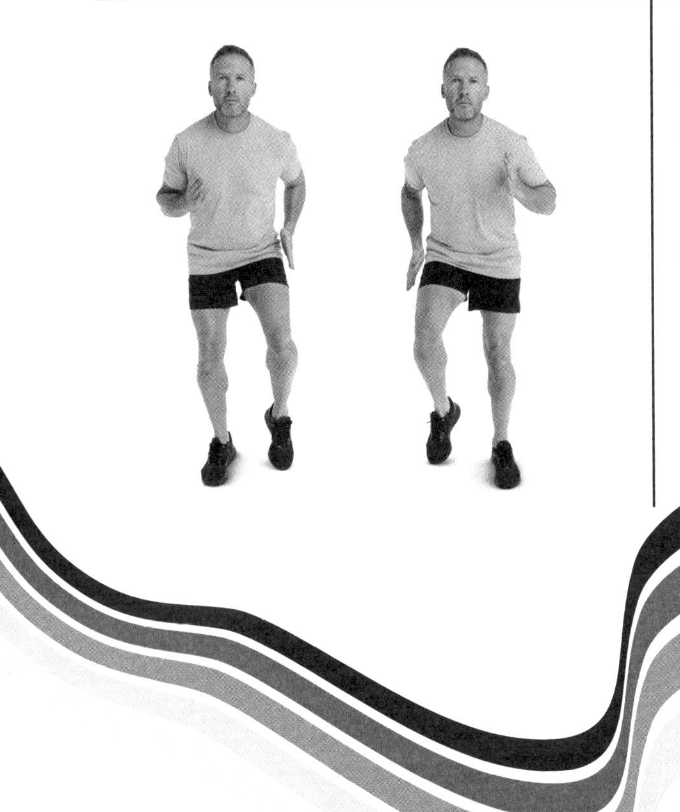

FAST FEET

1. **START POSITION:** Start in a standing position with your feet hip-width apart. Run on the spot, landing lightly on the balls of your feet, keeping your knees low while pumping your arms.
2. Keep your core engaged and legs moving as you continue to run on the spot.

CHALLENGE 11
TOP & TAIL

- **Let's top and tail some upper body work with some powerful moves to get the heart rate up and our muscles singing.**
- **Do each exercise 20 times. Then repeat each set 15, 10 then 5 times.**

BURPEES

1. **START POSITION:** Stand feet shoulder-width apart.
2. Bend your knees and reach forwards to place your hands on the floor.
3. Kick both legs straight out behind you into a high plank position.
4. Hop your legs back under your body and jump straight up into the air, reaching your arms overhead. Land with your knees slightly bent.

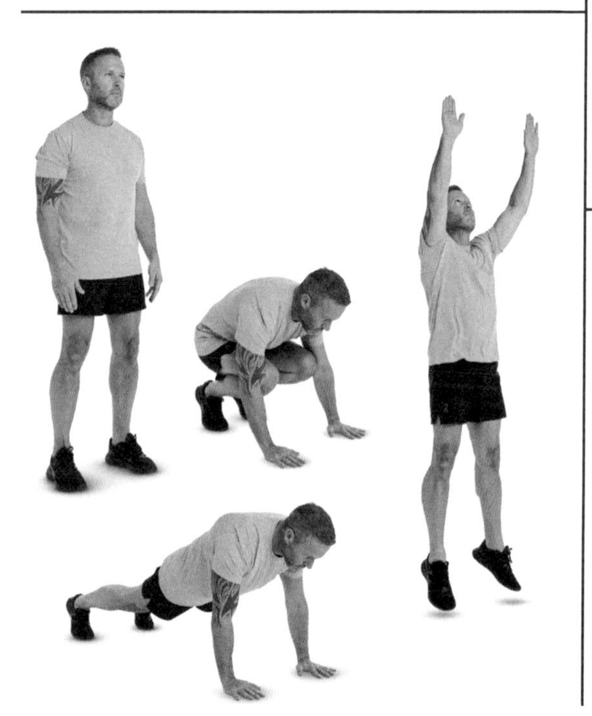

CLEAN AND PRESS (LEFT & RIGHT)

1. **START POSITION:** Stand with your feet hip-width apart with the kettlebell between your feet, turned sideways. Bend down and grip the kettlebell at the end of the handle with your right hand.
2. Drive through your glutes to stand up and bring the kettlebell up so it's resting on the outside of your forearm. Slightly bend your knees, keeping your chest upright.
3. Push the kettlebell up overhead as you drive up through your glutes to standing. Swap hands and repeat on the opposite side.

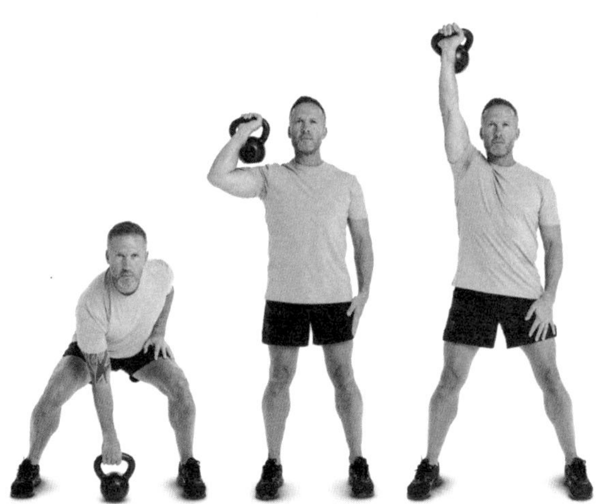

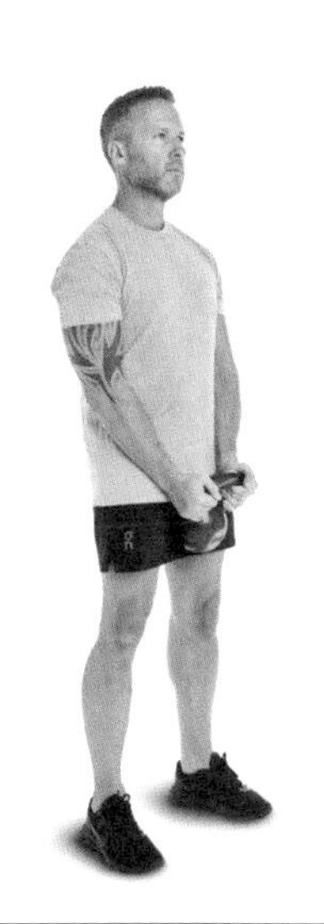
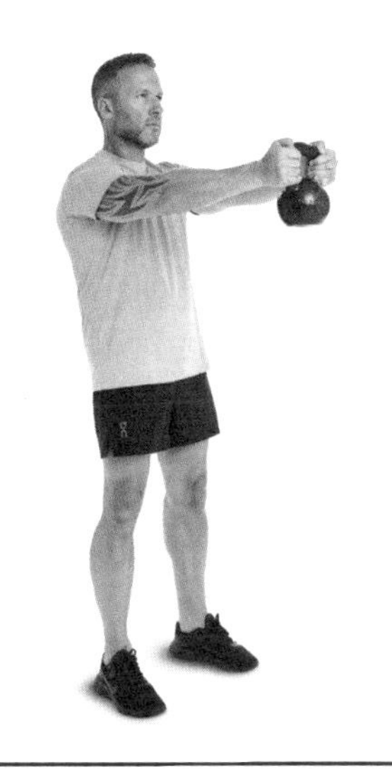

FRONT LATERAL RAISE

1. **START POSITION:** Stand with your feet shoulder-width apart, holding the kettlebell by the horns with both hands, palms facing each other and arms extended.
2. Raise the kettlebell to shoulder height without locking the elbows, lower with control and repeat.

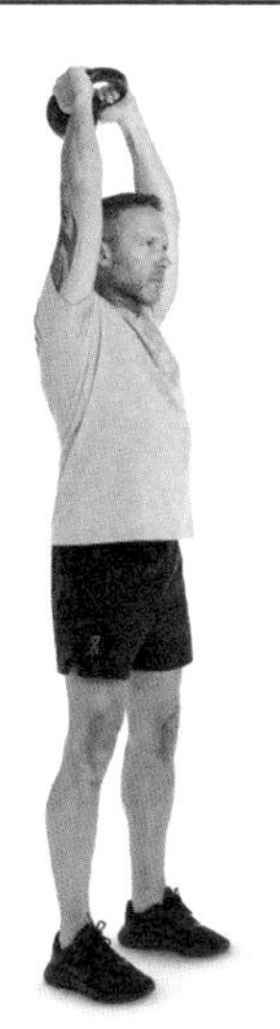
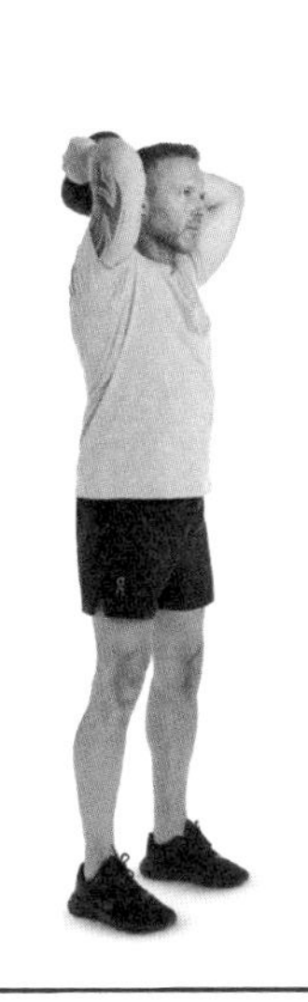

OVERHEAD TRICEP EXTENSIONS

1. **START POSITION:** Stand with your feet shoulder-width apart holding the kettlebell reverse grip by the horns above the head.
2. Lower the kettlebell with control behind your head, keeping your elbows facing forwards. Push the kettlebell back overhead to the starting position and repeat.

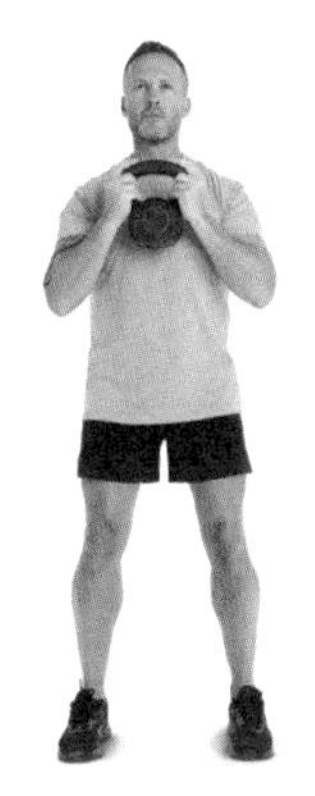
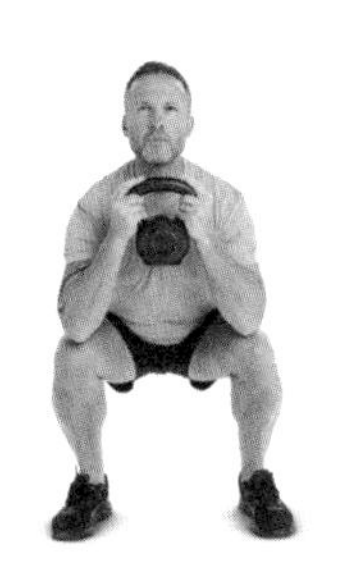

GOBLET SQUATS

1. **START POSITION:** Stand with your feet shoulder-width apart. Hold the kettlebell in front of your chest by the sides of the handle. Tuck your elbows in.
2. Keeping your back straight and core engaged, push your hips back and squat down, as if sitting down into a chair. Drive your weight through the heels to push back to a standing position.

INDEX

Note: page numbers in **bold** refer to illustrations.

PUBLISHERS ACKNOWLEDGMENTS
DK would like to thank Nicola Hodgson for copyediting, Nikki Dupin for design, Nicola Graimes for proofreading, and Lisa Footitt for indexing. DK would also like to thank Greenwich Peninsula for allowing us to use their location for photography.

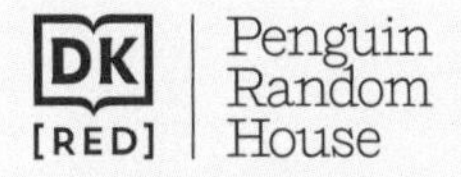

DK LONDON
Editorial Director Cara Armstrong
Project Editor Izzy Holton
Senior Designer Tania Gomes
Production Editor David Almond
Production Controller Kariss Ainsworth
Art Director Maxine Pedliham

Editorial Nicola Hodgson
Design Studio Nic&Lou
Photography David Cummings
Food Photography Vanessa Polignano
Food Stylist Susanna Unsworth
Assistant Food Stylist Lu Cottle
Prop Stylist Faye Wears

First published in Great Britain in 2024 by
DK RED, an imprint of Dorling Kindersley Limited
20 Vauxhall Bridge Road, London SW1V 2SA

The authorised representative in the EEA is
Dorling Kindersley Verlag GmbH. Arnulfstr. 124,
80636 Munich, Germany

The publisher would like to thank the following for their kind permission to reproduce their photograph:
Shutterstock.com: KADIVAR07 (Background image) used on pages 8-9, 15, 31, 33, 163.

10 9 8 7 6 5 4 3 2 1
001-339719-Dec/2024

A CIP catalogue record for this book is available from the British Library. ISBN: 978-0-2416-6169-7

Printed and bound in Slovakia

www.dk.com

This book was made with Forest Stewardship Council™ certified paper – one small step in DK's commitment to a sustainable future.
For more information go to www.dk.com/our-green-pledge

YOUR TRANSFORMATIONS

All these results were achieved in just 75 days.

BEFORE

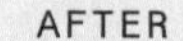

Josh Dyers

"What an experience! The Six Pack Revolution was the exact motivation I needed to turn things around. I never would have thought I could lose the fat and look so fit and strong while eating delicious meals and doing all my fitness from home! It gave me the confidence that every young person should have about their physique and mental state. The team at SPR make you feel very welcome and give you all the support you need to get it done from start to finish!"

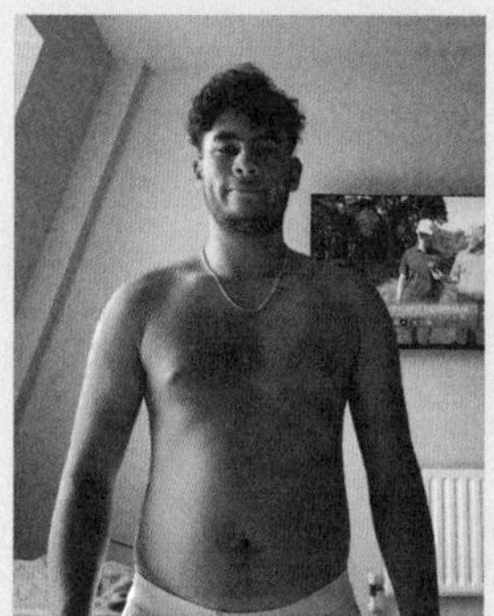

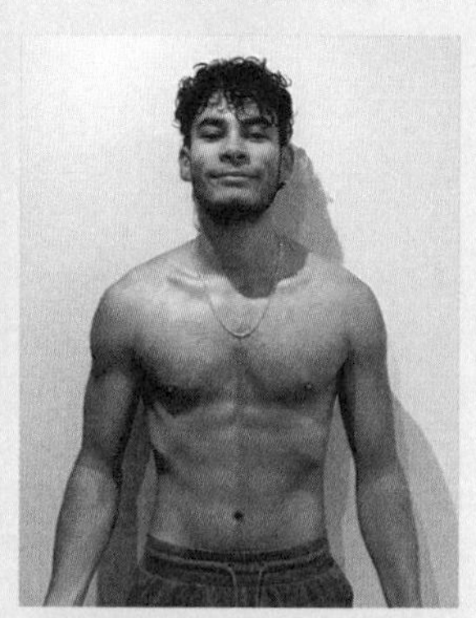

Sonny Dionisio

"My journey with SPR has been nothing short of transformative. I joined the March 2024 wave with a firm resolve to improve my fitness, eating habits, and overall health. Before joining, I struggled with hypertension and high cholesterol. After completing the program, not only did I achieve a six-pack (an unexpected bonus!), but more importantly, my health issues were resolved. The magic of the programme lies in its personalized approach and the approach and the supportive community it fosters. With tailored nutrition and workout plans, combined with expert guidance from the coaches, I surpassed my original goals and then some."

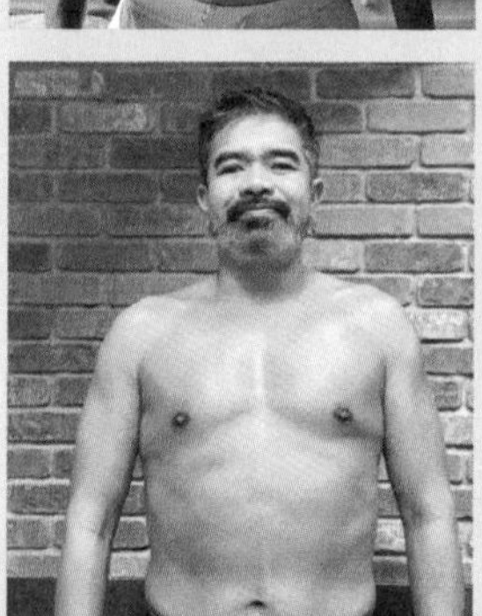

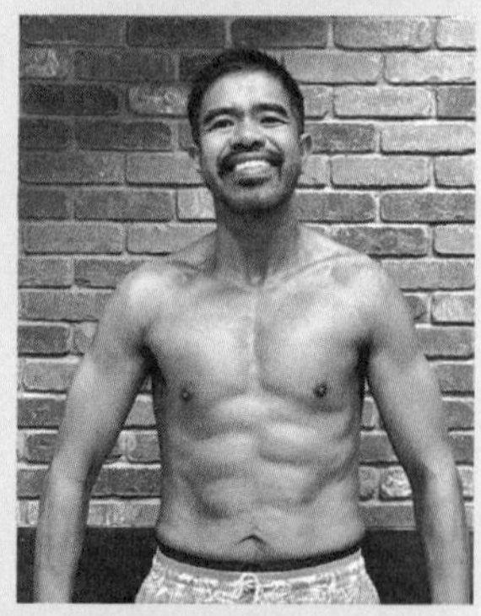

Sarah Holland

"Having been bigger for most of my adult life I was sceptical that this programme would work for me, but it has honestly changed my life and outlook towards food, drink and myself. I am now the fittest I have been in a very long while and I've even started running and will be taking part in my local half marathon in February. Thanks so much for everything, The Six Pack Revolution is a game changer."

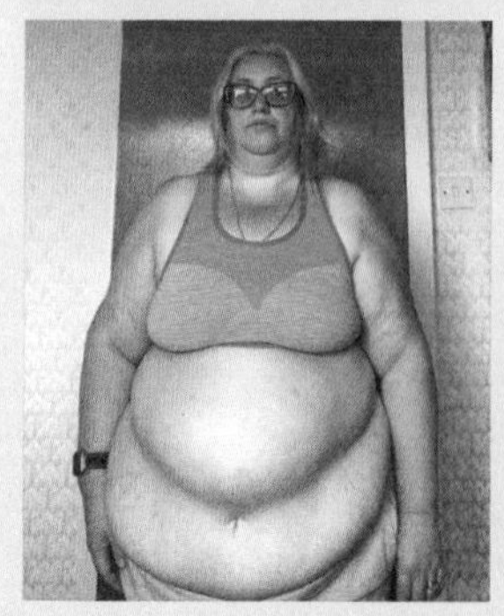

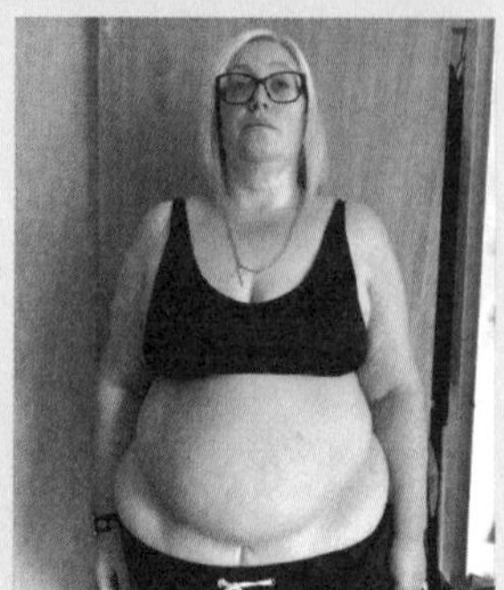

BEFORE AFTER

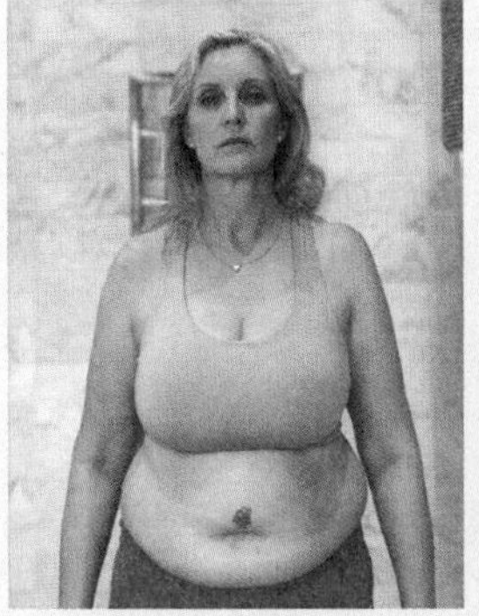

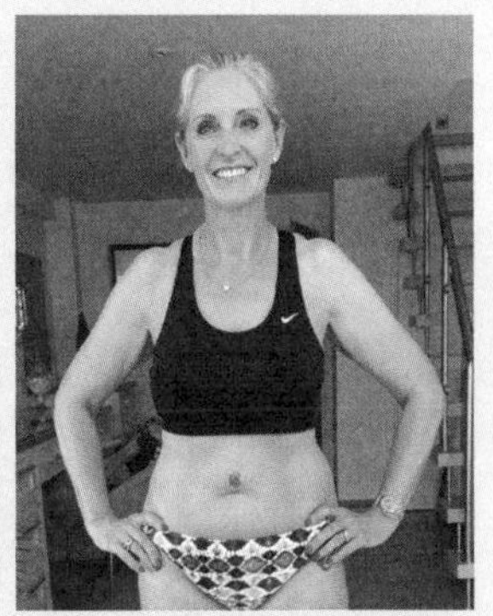

Claire Fernyhough

"As someone who has always been health conscious, I'd become overweight, self-conscious, self-doubting, and miserable, with aches and pains and injuries – I needed a kick up the behind, which The Six Pack Revolution figuratively did! Since doing the 'signature' programme, I'm a different person, I'm getting back to being 'me'. Not only did I lose body fat, the challenges pushed my physical abilities, developing muscle-tone, making me stronger physically and emotionally."

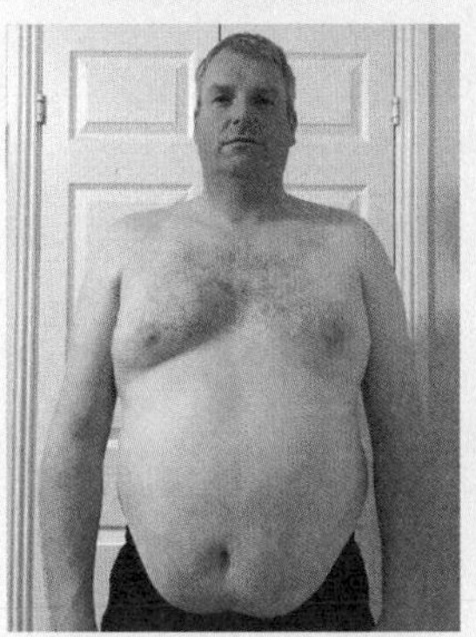

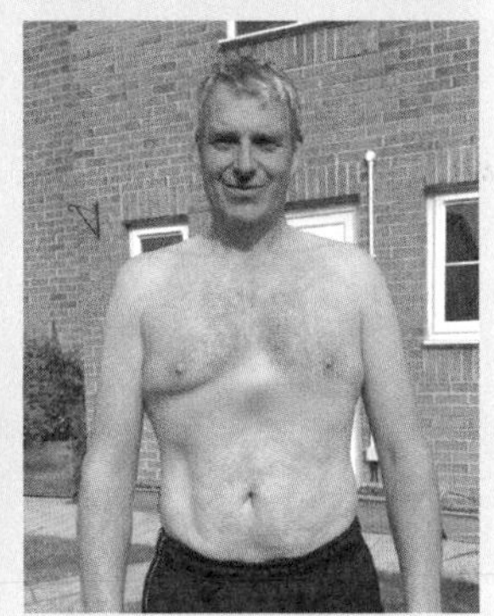

Gordon Steele

"Prior to starting the programme, I was overweight and unhappy with my life. My blood pressure was high and my doctors were convinced I was diabetic. After the first four weeks I had my blood sugars taken and they had dramatically fallen and the doctors said to hold off for another month on having to take any medication. After 75 days, I lost a considerable amount of weight, I felt great both mentally and physically. I had my blood sugar taken and to the doctors surprise I was back to normal, my blood pressure was also in perfect levels.

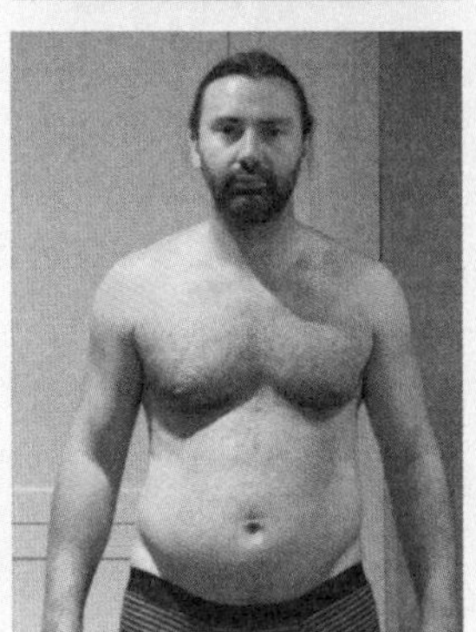

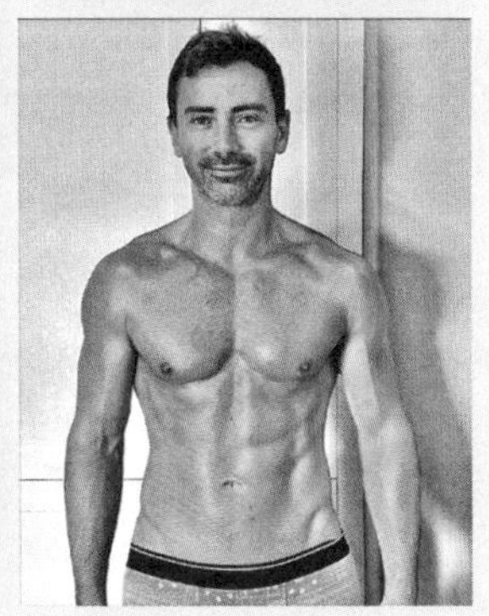

David Smith

"I joined The Six Pack Revolution because I'd let myself go a bit and the dad bod was creeping up on me. I was eating and drinking all the wrong things, feeling sluggish and just wasn't myself. The programme changed all of that for me and I found it actually really doable! And the result was, not only did I look like a superhero I felt like one too and was finally back to myself again, full of energy, strong, and happy."

THE EXPERTS

VICTORIA HARRISON
Nutritionist

DR AGGY YORK
MBChB, MRC GP

DR JODIE BOOTH
Doctor of Biochemistry BSc,PhD, CSSM Dip, MISRM

KAREN SCHRANZ
Psychotherapist

DR. MIGUEL GUITTEREZ
Chiropractor MChiro. S.T.R. Bio Mechanical Expert

THANK YOU

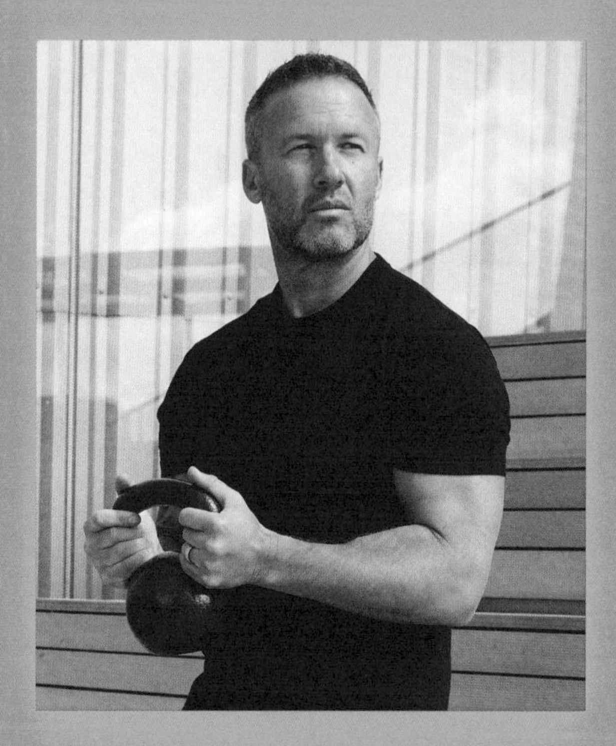

Well, here we are at the end of my second book, *High Protein Meals In Minutes*, and what a journey it's been. I need to thank every participant that has taken part in this life-changing programme over the years and embraced the SPR way of life. It has been an honour to walk by your side and watch you change your lives physically, mentally, and emotionally. Every single one of you is a true inspiration and you should all be proud of yourselves for working hard for a healthier, happier life. Thank you for your contribution, your support, your love for the programme and for glimpsing the magic of life through the eyes of The Six Pack Revolution! I must thank everyone that has sent me such touching, heartfelt messages about how I have changed and saved their lives. Not just physically and aesthetically, but in the way the programme has had a serious impact on their health, mental health and positive attitude to themselves and those around them. The truth is, however, that it's you that made those changes and we just gave you the tools to implement them.

I have a world-class team of experts in Victoria, Aggy, Karen, Jodie, and Miguel, who share their knowledge and guidance with me. My global team of motivational coaches also work tirelessly to make sure that each and every one of you experience the magic of The Six Pack Revolution. Team – your dedication and devotion to the programme and its participants is beyond all expectations. I will never be able to thank you enough and am truly grateful.

Of course, I would like to thank my family; my wife and best friend, Victoria, my children, Scarlett, Hugo and Jasper for sharing me with my work and for giving me the beautiful loving home support that I desperately need. Thank you, as ever, to my parents for instilling values in me to always work hard and to follow my passion and for being the best parents and grandparents anyone could ever ask for.

My right-hand woman Sam who literally does everything for me and my amazing management team Annie and Sarah. We work so closely together as a family and continue to strive for a better life for everyone that comes through our programme.

To Paul "Piqué" King, I thank you for allowing me to bounce my ideas off you, drive you mad with what floods into my head and always return to me with a voice of reason and logic.

I would like to give a huge thank you to Tom Kirby for assisting me in creating these delicious meals. Tom trained at the Savoy London, is now the head team chef to the England Rugby squad.

Vanessa Polignano, once again your stunning food photography has hit the spot and it's been a pleasure to work with you over these years. I would like to thank Elizabeth Bullen, who adds glitter to my written word

Finally, I would like to express my gratitude to everyone at DK, with a special nod to Cara, Izzy, and Tania for their time and patience in helping me complete this book. A shout-out to David who seamlessly manages to make me look handsome and catches my "best side" in every photo. It is always a pleasure and inspiring to collaborate with you.

To all those who have not experienced the life-changing effects of The Six Pack Revolution yet, I am looking forward to seeing you soon. It's going to blow your mind and change your life forever! Wishing you all the love and luck in the world.